Protein Kinases - Promising Targets for Anticancer Drug Research

Edited by Rajesh Kumar Singh

Published in London, United Kingdom

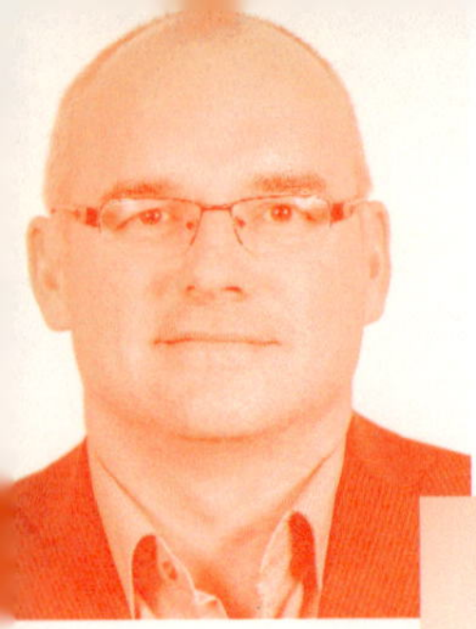
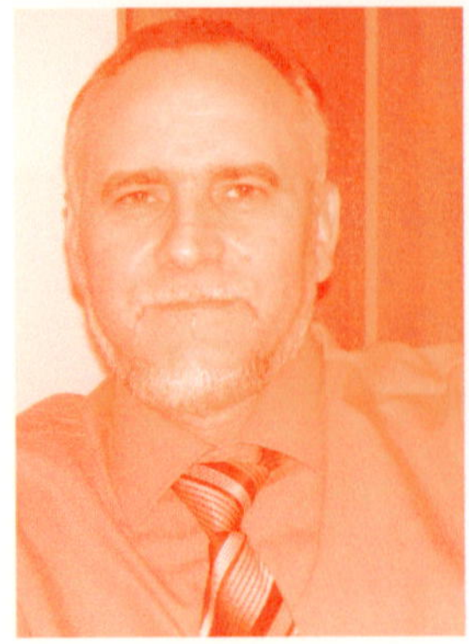
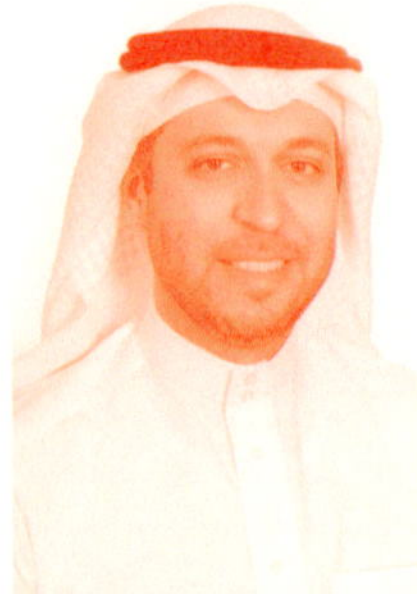
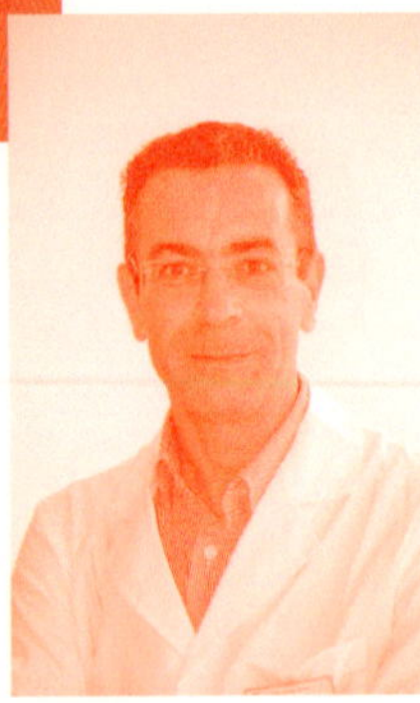
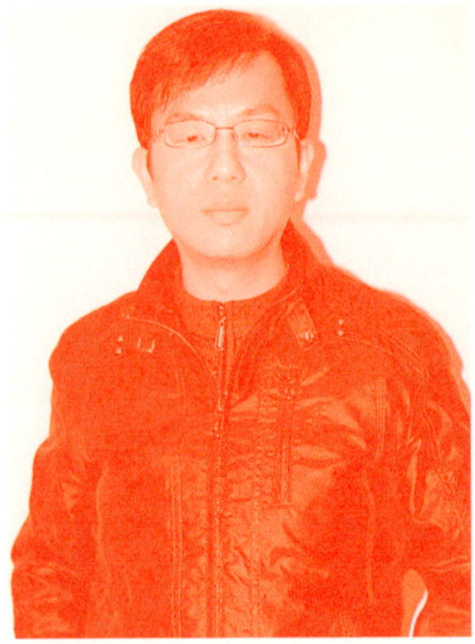
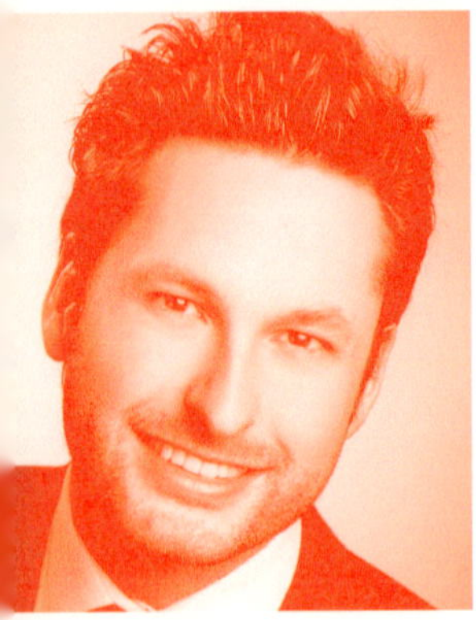
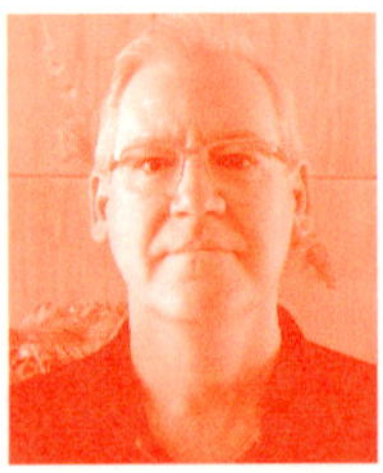

IntechOpen

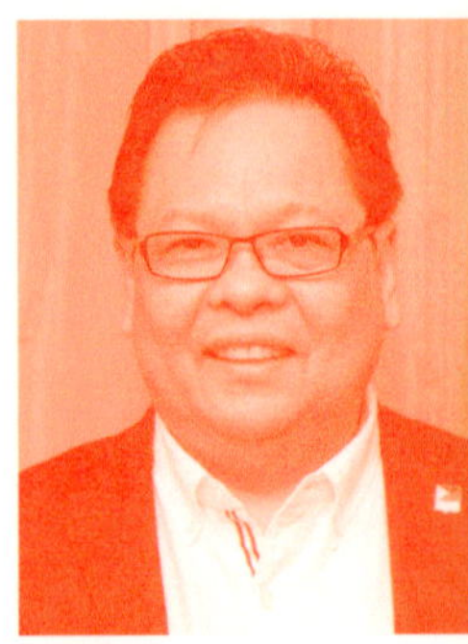
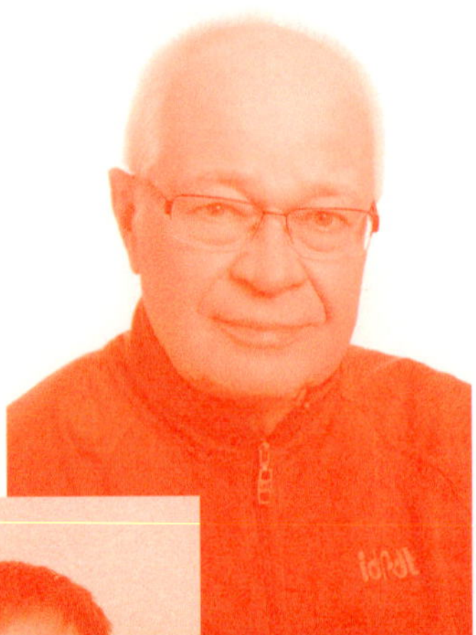
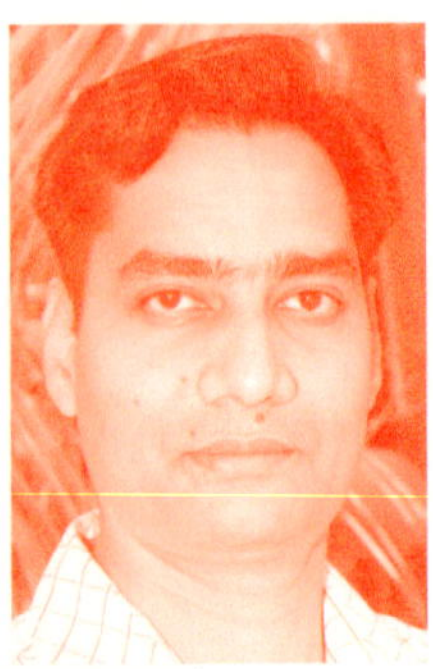
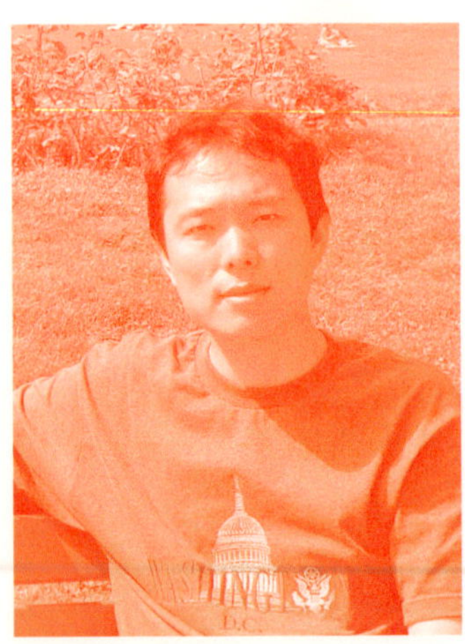
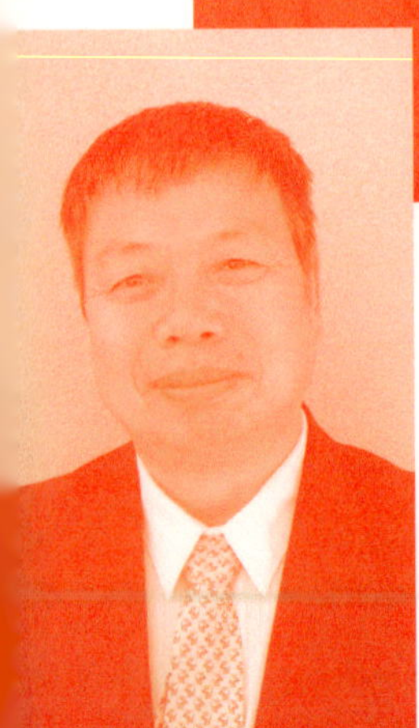
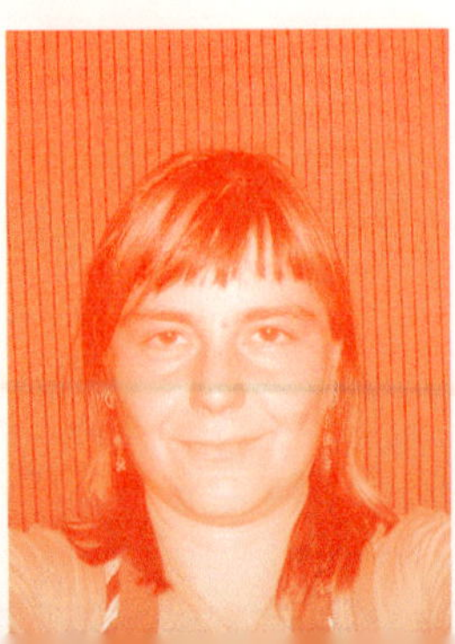

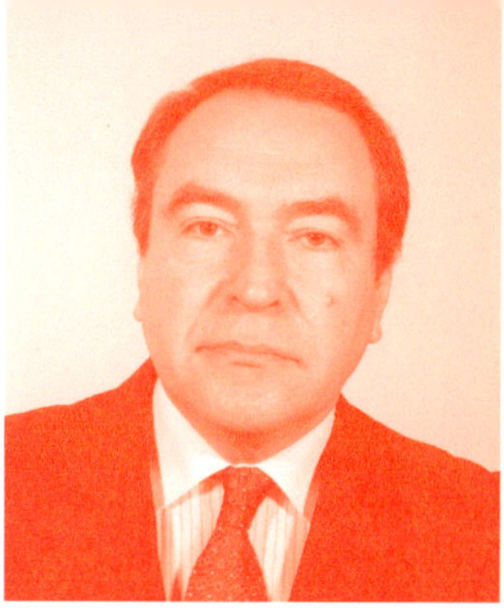
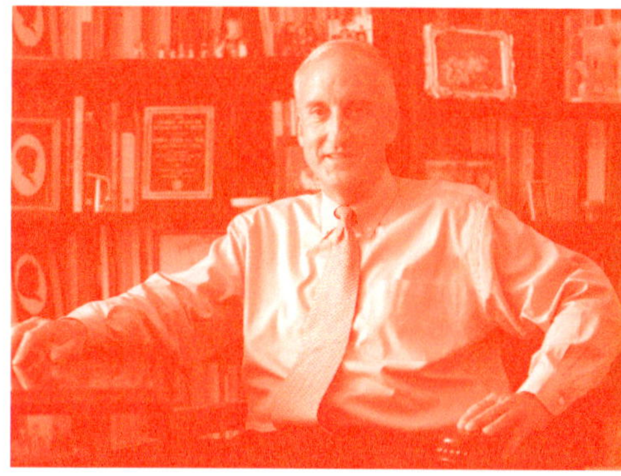
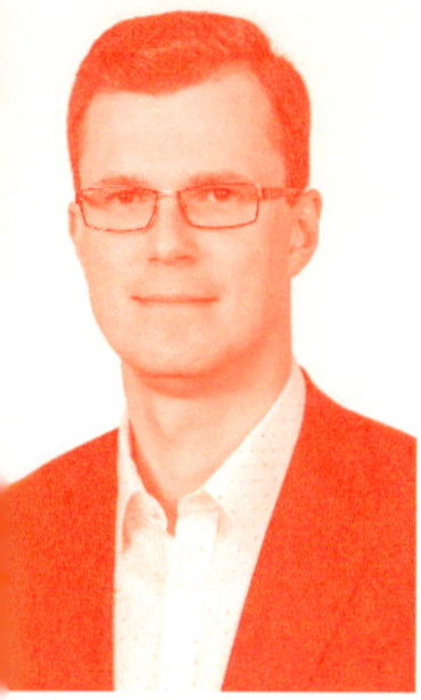
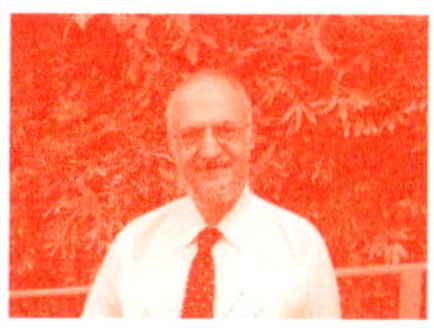
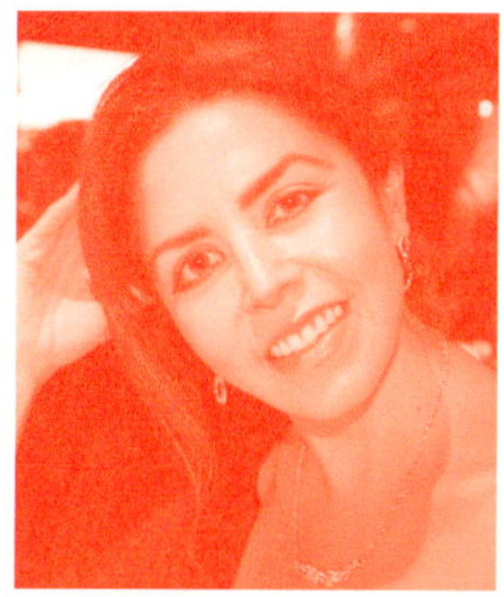

Supporting open minds since 2005

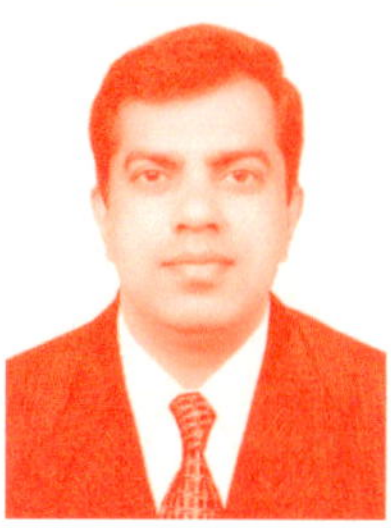
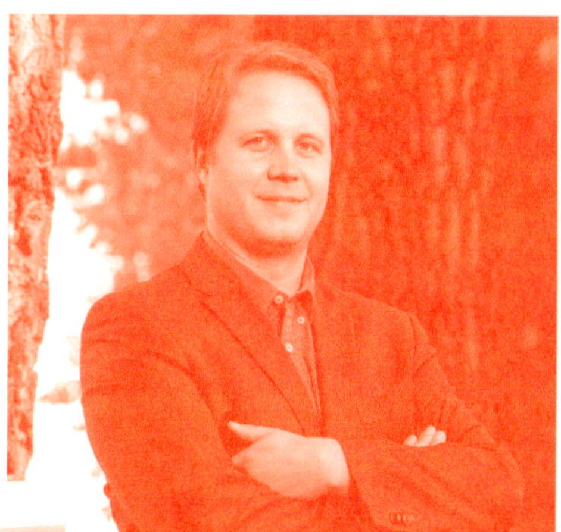
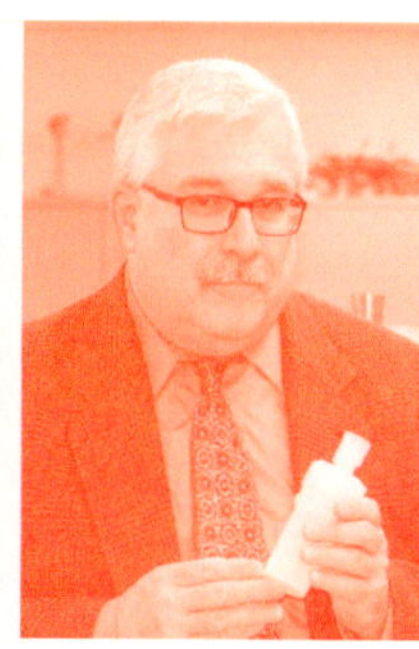
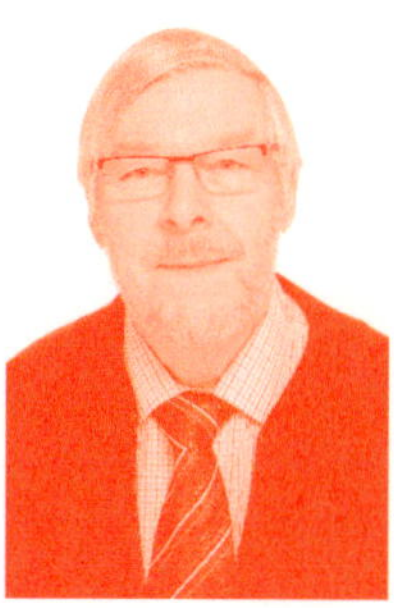
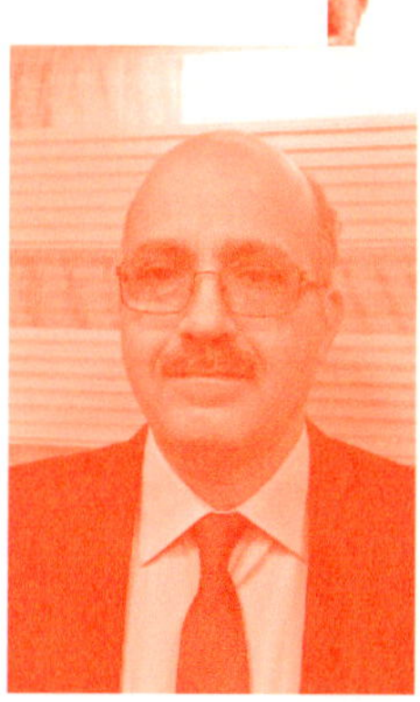
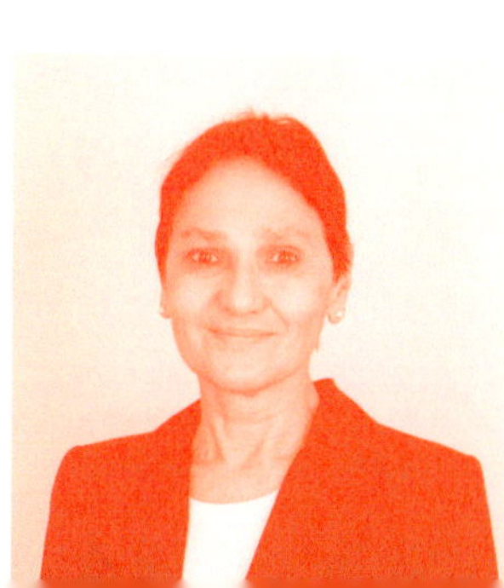
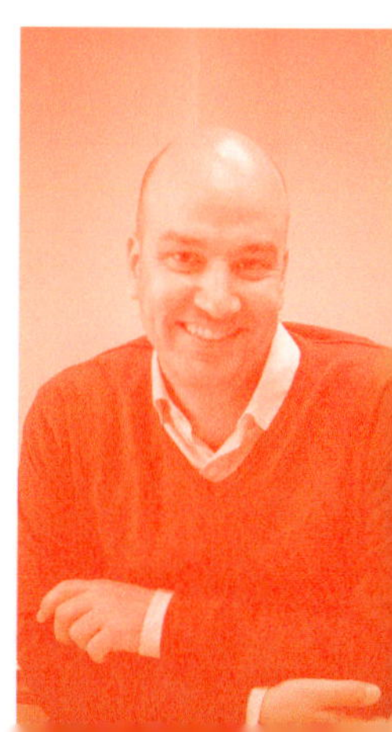

Protein Kinases - Promising Targets for Anticancer Drug Research
http://dx.doi.org/10.5772/intechopen.82939
Edited by Rajesh Kumar Singh

Contributors
Sangwook Wu, Sungmin Lee, Suhyun Park, Hyun Jung Yoon, Philip E. Bourne, Zheng Zhao, Hülya Ayar Kayali, Esra Bulut Atalay, Elçin Çağatay, Seminay Güler, Duygu Erdoğan, Gizem Kurşunluoğlu, Yonca Güngör, Panneerselvam Theivendren, Selvaraj Kunjiappan, Murugananthan Gopal, Yashoda Mariappa Hegde, Senthil Rajan Dhramalingam, Sivakumar Vellaichamy, Sattanathan Kumar, Moran Grossman, Elaine Adler, Somi Patranabis, Rajesh Kumar Singh, Rohit Bhatia

First published in London, United Kingdom, 2021 by IntechOpen
IntechOpen is the global imprint of INTECHOPEN LIMITED, registered in England and Wales, registration number: 11086078, 5 Princes Gate Court, London, SW7 2QJ, United Kingdom
Printed in Croatia

British Library Cataloguing-in-Publication Data
A catalogue record for this book is available from the British Library

Additional hard and PDF copies can be obtained from orders@intechopen.com

Protein Kinases - Promising Targets for Anticancer Drug Research
Edited by Rajesh Kumar Singh
p. cm.

This title is part of the Biochemistry Book Series, Volume 24
Topic: Proteomics
Series Editor: Miroslav Blumenberg
Topic Editors: Paolo Iadarola and Simona Viglio

Print ISBN 978-1-83880-906-5
Online ISBN 978-1-83880-907-2
eBook (PDF) ISBN 978-1-83880-908-9
ISSN 2632-0983

For EU product safety concerns:
IN TECH d.o.o., Prolaz Marije Krucifikse Kozulić 3, 51000 Rijeka, Croatia, info@intechopen.com or visit our website at intechopen.com.

IntechOpen Book Series

Biochemistry

Volume 24

Aims and Scope of the Series

Biochemistry, the study of chemical transformations occurring within living organisms, impacts all of the life sciences, from molecular crystallography and genetics, to ecology, medicine and population biology. Biochemistry studies macromolecules - proteins, nucleic acids, carbohydrates and lipids –their building blocks, structures, functions and interactions. Much of biochemistry is devoted to enzymes, proteins that catalyze chemical reactions, enzyme structures, mechanisms of action and their roles within cells. Biochemistry also studies small signaling molecules, coenzymes, inhibitors, vitamins and hormones, which play roles in the life process. Biochemical experimentation, besides coopting the methods of classical chemistry, e.g., chromatography, adopted new techniques, e.g., X-ray diffraction, electron microscopy, NMR, radioisotopes, and developed sophisticated microbial genetic tools, e.g., auxotroph mutants and their revertants, fermentation, etc. More recently, biochemistry embraced the 'big data' omics systems.
Initial biochemical studies have been exclusively analytic: dissecting, purifying and examining individual components of a biological system; in exemplary words of Efraim Racker, (1913 –1991) "Don't waste clean thinking on dirty enzymes." Today, however, biochemistry is becoming more agglomerative and comprehensive, setting out to integrate and describe fully a particular biological system. The 'big data' metabolomics can define the complement of small molecules, e.g., in a soil or biofilm sample; proteomics can distinguish all the proteins comprising e.g., serum; metagenomics can identify all the genes in a complex environment e.g., the bovine rumen. This Biochemistry Series will address both the current research on biomolecules, and the emerging trends with great promise.

Meet the Series Editor

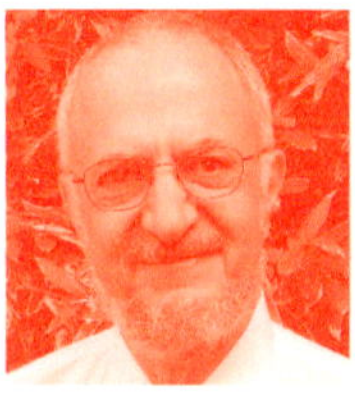

Miroslav Blumenberg, Ph.D., was born in Subotica and received his BSc in Belgrade, Yugoslavia. He completed his Ph.D. at MIT in Organic Chemistry; he followed up his Ph.D. with two post-doctoral study periods at Stanford University. Since 1983, he has been a faculty member of the RO Perelman Department of Dermatology, NYU School of Medicine, where he is codirector of a training grant in cutaneous biology. Dr. Blumenberg's research is focused on the epidermis, expression of keratin genes, transcription profiling, keratinocyte differentiation, inflammatory diseases and cancers, and most recently the effects of the microbiome on the skin. He has published more than 100 peer-reviewed research articles and graduated numerous Ph.D. and postdoctoral students.

Meet the Volume Editor

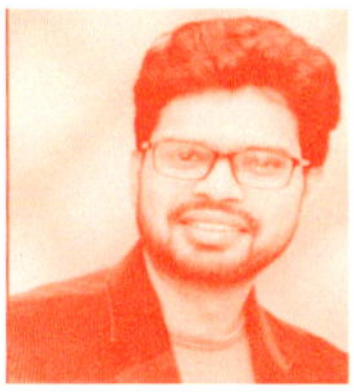

Dr. Singh received a BPharm (2003) and MPharm (2005) from Panjab University, Chandigarh, India, and a Ph.D. (2013) from Punjab Technical University (PTU), Jalandhar, India. He has more than sixteen years of teaching experience and has supervised numerous postgraduate and Ph.D. students. He has to his credit more than seventy papers in SCI- and SCOPUS-indexed journals, fifty-five conference proceedings, four books, six Best Paper Awards, and five projects from different government agencies. He is currently an editorial board member of eight international journals and a reviewer for more than fifty scientific journals. He received Top Reviewer and Excellent Peer Reviewer Awards from Publons in 2016 and 2017, respectively. He is also on the panel of The International Reviewer for reviewing research proposals for grants from the Royal Society. He also serves as a Publons Academy mentor and Bentham brand ambassador.

Contents

Preface

Exploring new cancer targets is integral for developing effective anticancer drugs. Protein kinase-driven phosphorylation is one of the vital mechanisms controlling intracellular signalling pathways that regulate many cellular processes, such as cell division, proliferation, growth, survival, and apoptosis. Alteration of different protein kinases can result in remarkable changes in these processes. Moreover, these protein kinases are frequently recognized as oncogenic and can be crucial for the survival and spread of cancer cells. Because of the fundamental role of protein kinases in cell biology and their function in numerous sarcomas and cancers, an intensive search for new kinase inhibitors in academia and industries has been enduring for the last two decades. This book includes seven chapters by leading researchers in the field that focus on protein kinase signalling pathways as a molecular drug target for anticancer drug design.

In Chapter 1, the authors summarize the progress in protein kinase targeted drug development against cancer over the last five years. Protein kinase has become the most imperative and commercial class of drug target, enticing pharmaceutical industries to spend 30% of their current research investments in developing kinase inhibitors for various therapeutic implications. This is exemplified by the fact that seventy-five drugs targeting protein kinase have been clinically approved to date. More than 100 kinase inhibitors are in the final stages of development and are likely to be approved in the coming years. Only about 10% of kinases have been studied extensively to date. Despite tremendous advancements in kinase drug development, many kinases are unexplored as of yet. The development of kinase inhibitors will be expected at the forefront of medicine for the foreseeable future.

Kinase-targeting drug design is challenging. It requires designing inhibitors that can bind to specific kinases when all kinase catalytic domains share a common folding scaffold that binds adenosine triphosphate (ATP). Thus, obtaining the desired selectivity, given the whole human kinome, is fundamental during early-stage drug discovery. Several protein kinase inhibitors have been developed in the last decade, but lack of selectivity and adverse toxicities resulted in the discontinuation of these promising drug candidates. But now, scientists are questing for selective kinase inhibitors to get rid of any unwanted toxicity. In this context, Chapters 2 and 3 are devoted to protein kinase selectivity. In Chapter 2, Grossman and Adler summarize the challenges and common toxicities of kinase inhibitors, management of associated toxicities, and different methodologies available for measuring and quantifying kinase inhibitor selectivity. It also discusses newly emerging inhibitors that are more selective and safer.

In Chapter 3, Zhao and Bourne work on deciphering and analyzing the kinase-ligand characteristic and structure-activity relationship and prioritizing the desired drug molecules across the whole kinome. To obtain the desired kinase selectivity, the complete human kinome was explored by in silico structure-based method synergistically with multiple cell-based or protein-based assay platforms such as KINOMEscan.

c-Src tyrosine kinase plays an essential role in signal transduction pathways, where its activity is regulated by phosphorylation of the two tyrosine residues. Chapter 4 by Sangwook Wu et al. perform targeted molecular dynamics simulation to obtain the trajectory of conformational transition of c-Src tyrosine kinase from inactive to active form using network analysis to time series of correlation among residues. Based on the analysis of the three centrality measures (betweenness, closeness, and degree), it was observed that Lys321 plays an essential role in the conformational transition of c-Src tyrosine kinase and may be another candidate for a switch for the conformational transition of c-Src tyrosine kinase.

Chapter 5 by Theivendren et al. discusses the function of protein kinases in signal transduction and their cellular signaling pathways with beautiful illustrations. This chapter delves into the catalytic domain of protein kinases, the effect of over-expression and the therapeutic roles of various protein kinase inhibitors. It also outlines a systematic method for hybrid therapies to solve the issue of protein kinase resistance.

Receptor tyrosine kinases (RTKs) are important molecules involved in regulating different cellular functions. Recently, RTKs have been extensively studied, as they are associated with different types of cancer and related diseases. Chapter 6 by Somi Patranabis presents recent advances and challenges in RTK-related research to obtain an overview of the problems and possibilities associated with targeted therapy. This chapter helps in deciphering novel therapeutic applications of RTKs in the future.

The dawn of protein kinase inhibitors in cancer therapy has led to a paradigm shift in treating cancer. So far, there are sixty-two FDA-approved therapeutic agents targeting different protein kinases, eight of which were approved in 2020. Chapter 7 by Hulya Ayar Kayali et al. focuses on kinases' role in oncogenic pathways and the kinase inhibitors targeting these pathways as a therapeutic option. These protein kinase inhibitors are grouped as growth factor receptor inhibitors, Ras/Raf/Mek inhibitors, phosphoinositide 3-kinase (PI3K), and cyclin-dependent kinase inhibitors with structures and mechanisms of action. It also describes other targets and agents such as protein kinase c and 3 phosphoinositide-dependent kinase 1.

I would like to thank all the contributors for their intricate and scholarly work. We are also grateful to Ms. Marijana Francetic at IntechOpen, who took over the management of the production of this book under the challenging circumstances of the COVID pandemic and whose contribution is much appreciated. We are confident that this book will be a compelling guide to facilitate researchers, pharmacologists, and medicinal chemists in understanding the mechanism of protein kinase, which can help develop new anticancer agents.

Rajesh Kumar Singh
Department of Pharmaceutical Chemistry,
Shivalik College of Pharmacy, Nangal,
IKG Punjab Technical University,
Jalandhar, Punjab,
India

Chapter 1

Introductory Chapter: Protein Kinases as Promising Targets for Drug Design against Cancer

Rohit Bhatia and Rajesh K. Singh

1. Introduction

Cancer is one of the most dreadful and highly prevailing life-threatening ailments of the modern age. Despite a great advancement in the health sector, still it is the leading cause of mortality around the globe [1, 2]. The continuous research is in progress for several years to design therapeutic agents against cancer with greater efficacy, specificity, and least toxicity. For the past two decades, the protein kinase family has been greatly focused by the researchers for drug development against cancer. There are about 538 protein kinase enzymes that are encoded by the human genome, which function mainly by transferring a γ-phosphate group from the ATP site toward amino acid residues such as serine, threonine, or tyrosine residues [3–5]. It is evident that several members of this protein kinase family have tendencies to initiate and develop human cancers [6, 7]. The recently developed small molecules as potential kinase inhibitors in the therapy of a variety of cancers have witnessed the significance of kinases as a target against cancers. Moreover, these are in second place as a target for drugs after the G-protein-coupled receptors [8]. Protein kinases are associated with the promotion of cell proliferation, migration, and survival and, when they are dysregulated/overexpressed, lead to oncogenesis [9, 10]. During the past decades, it has been observed that human malignancies are largely associated with modulation or dysfunction of protein and lipid kinases due to the deactivation of phosphatases resulting from chromosomal abnormalities or mutations [11, 12]. It is worth notable that the anti-inflammatory kinases such as EGFR, VEGFR, BCR-ABL, ALK, KIT, HER2, and several others are involved in the development of solid cancers including chronic lymphoid leukemia, lymphoblastic leukemia, mantle cell lymphoma, myelogenous lymphoma, and several other types of cancers [13]. These kinases show a pro-tumor effect associated with loss of normal kinase functioning followed by mutations and associations with high-regulatory T cell pathogens [14]. These pathogens ultimately activate the anti-inflammatory kinases and initiate the development of solid cancers. The role of some kinases in the development of cancers has been depicted in **Figure 1**.

Kinase amplifications are able to play diagnostic, prognostic, therapeutic as well as biomarker roles in cancer [15]. The amplifications of EGFR have been well seen in a variety of cancers including non-small cell lung cancer, colorectal cancer, bladder cancer, pancreatic, and breast cancer, whereas ERBB2 amplifications are associated with esophageal, gastric, breast, and ovarian cancers [16–18]. Overexpression of EGFR, ERBB2, EPHA2, and AKT2 are the best examples of biomarkers for cancers [19, 20].

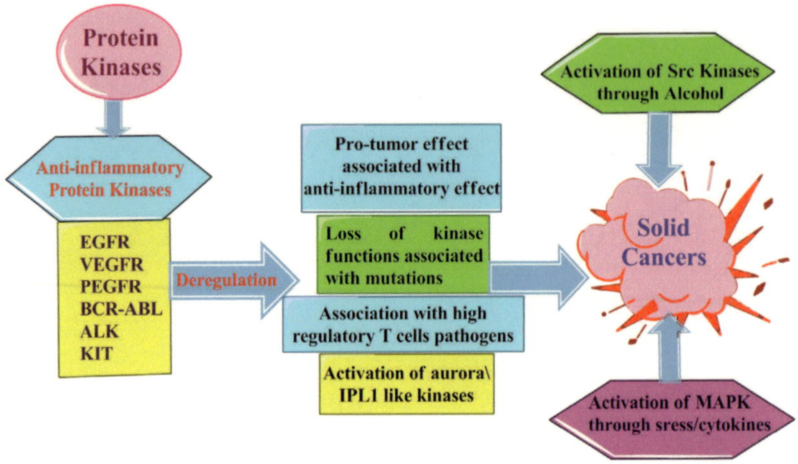

Figure 1.
Impact of protein kinases in development of cancer.

2. Progress in the development of protein kinase inhibitors against cancer

In the past two decades, there has been a remarkable progress made in the drug development process involving protein kinases as a target. The first FDA approved drug imatinib was launched in 2001 against chronic myeloid leukemia which inhibits Abelson (ABL) tyrosine kinase [21]. It was proved to be a blockbuster drug with polypharmacological effects. From 2001 to 2021, in a span of 20 years, there has been an extraordinary progress made with the discovery of more potent and specific small-molecule kinase inhibitors and about 70 new drugs have got approval in this time span [22]. These drugs have left a promising positive impact to improve the drug design strategies and therapy to treat the cancers and conditions associated with it. **Table 1** comprises the details of kinase inhibitor drugs approved by the FDA from 2015 to 2021 [23–58].

The modern strategies adopted for the development of selective kinase inhibitors include synthesis along with structure-based design approaches facilitated by molecular docking, crystallographic studies, and NMR spectroscopy [59]. It is surprising that alone USA has filed more than 10 thousand patent applications for kinase inhibitors since 2001. Beyond the discovery of small-molecule kinase inhibitors, kinase-targeted antibodies have also been postulated against different cancers such as cetuximab (colorectal, head, and neck cancer), trastuzumab (breast cancer) [60]. Various small-molecule kinase inhibitors have different inhibitory modes and on the basis of these modes, these inhibitors have been divided into five categories (**Figure 2**). Type I inhibitors contain a heterocyclic moiety in their structure to occupy purine binding pocket and serves as a template for side chains to occupy the hydrophobic region. These inhibitors are basically ATP-binding site competitors and mimic the purine ring of ATP. These bind to the active conformational side and cause alteration of structural conformation [61]. Type II inhibitors target the inactive conformation and occupy the catalytic region of the unphosphorylated inactive conformation. These kinases explore the new binding patterns in the hydrophobic pocket associated with conformational changes of phenylalanine residue of the Asp-Phe-Gly (DFG) system [62]. Type III inhibitors are regarded as allosteric inhibitors and exhibit their action *via* binding to the outer catalytic ATP-binding site and alter kinase activity in an allosteric

S. No.	Drug	Brand name	Year of approval	Inhibitory target	Indication	References
1.	Palbociclib	Ibrance	2015	CDK4/6 inhibitor	Advanced metastatic breast cancer	[23]
2.	Lenvatinib	Lenvima	2015	VEGFR1/2/3 inhibitor	Progressive/ differentiated thyroid cancer	[24]
3.	Cobimetinib	Cotellic	2015	MEK inhibitor	Melanoma	[25]
4.	Osimertinib	Tagrisso	2015	EGFR inhibitor	Non-small cell lung carcinomas with specific mutations	[26]
5.	Necitumumab	Portrazza	2015	EGFR antibody	Advanced (metastatic) squamous non-small cell lung cancer	[27]
6.	Alectinib	Alecensa	2015	ALK inhibitor	Non-small cell lung cancer	[28]
7.	Olaratumab	Lartruvo	2016	PDGFRA inhibitor	Soft tissue sarcoma	[29]
8.	Ribociclib	Kisqali	2016	CDK4/6 inhibitor	Advanced breast cancer	[30]
9.	Brigatinib	Alunbrig	2017	ALK and EGFR inhibitor	Non-small cell lung cancer	[31]
10.	Copanlisib	Aliqopa	2017	PI3K inhibitor	Relapsed follicular lymphoma	[32]
11.	Abemaciclib	Verzenio	2017	CDK4/6 inhibitors	Advanced metastatic breast cancer	[33]
12.	Acalabrutinib	Calquence	2017	BTK inhibitor	Mantle cell lymphoma	[34]
13.	Binimetinib	Mektovi	2018	MEK inhibitor	Unresectable or metastatic melanoma	[35]
14.	Encorafenib	Braftovi	2018	MEK inhibitor	Unresectable or metastatic melanoma	[36]
15.	Duvelisib	Copiktra	2018	PI3K inhibitor	Refractory chronic lymphocytic leukemia, small lymphocytic lymphoma, and follicular lymphoma	[37]
16.	Dacomitinib	Vizimpro	2018	EGFR inhibitor	Metastatic non-small cell lung cancer	[38]
17.	Lorlatinib	Lorbrena	2018	ALK and ROS1 inhibitor	Metastatic non-small cell lung cancer	[39]
18.	Gilteritinib	Xospata	2018	AXL inhibitor	Relapsed or refractory acute myeloid leukemia	[40]
19.	Erdafitinib	Balversa	2019	FGFR inhibitor	Locally advanced or metastatic bladder cancer	[41]
20.	Alpelisib	Piqray	2019	PI3K inhibitor	Breast cancer	[42]
21.	Pexidartinib	Turalio	2019	inhibitor of CSF1, KIT, and FLT3	Symptomatic tenosynovial giant cell tumor	[43]

S. No.	Drug	Brand name	Year of approval	Inhibitory target	Indication	References
22.	Entrectinib	Rozlytrek	2019	inhibitor of ALK, ROS1, TKI, and TRKA/B/C	Metastatic non-small cell lung cancer	[44]
23.	Zanubrutinib	Brukinsa	2019	BTK inhibitor	Mantle cell lymphoma	[45]
24.	Avapritinib	Ayvakit	2020	PDGFRA receptor kinase inhibitor	Metastatic gastrointestinal stromal tumors	[46]
25.	Selumetinib	Koselugo	2020	BRAF kinase inhibitor	Neurofibromatosis type I	[47]
26.	Tucatinib	Tukyssa	2020	EBBR2 inhibitor	Metastatic HER2-positive breast cancer	[48]
27.	Pemigatinib	Pemazyre	2020	FGFR2 inhibitor	Advanced/metastatic or surgically unresectable cholangiocarcinoma	[49]
28.	Capmatinib	Tabrecta	2020	MET kinase inhibitor	Metastatic non-small cell lung cancer	[50]
29.	Selpercatinib	Retevmo	2020	RET receptor kinase	Non-small cell lung cancer, metastatic medullary thyroid cancer, or advanced or metastatic thyroid cancer	[51]
30.	Ripretinib	Qinlock	2020	PDGFRA and KIT receptor kinase inhibitor	Gist	[52]
31.	Pralsetinib	Gavreto	2020	RET receptor kinase inhibitor	Thyroid cancer, non-small cell lung cancer	[53]
32.	Margetuximab	Margenza	2020	HER2 inhibitor	HER2-positive breast cancer	[54]
33.	Trilaciclib	Cosela	2021	CDK4/6 inhibitor	Extensive-stage small cell lung cancer	[55]
34.	Infigratinib	Truseltiq	2021	FGFR2 inhibitor	Cholangiocarcinomas with FGFR2 fusion proteins	[56]
35.	Tepotinib	Tepmetco	2021	Met Kinase	Met mutation-positive non-small cell lung carcinoma	[57]
36.	Tivozanib	Fotvida	2021	VEGFR2 inhibitor	Renal cell carcinoma	[58]

Table 1.
FDA-approved kinase inhibitors against various cancers during 2015–2021.

way. Type IV kinase inhibitors are regarded as substrate-directed inhibitors and undergo reversible binding outside the ATP pocket. These are non-competitive inhibitors and do not compete with ATP [63]. Type V inhibitors are covalent inhibitors and bind through an irreversible covalent bond to catalytic nucleophilic cysteine active site of the enzyme.

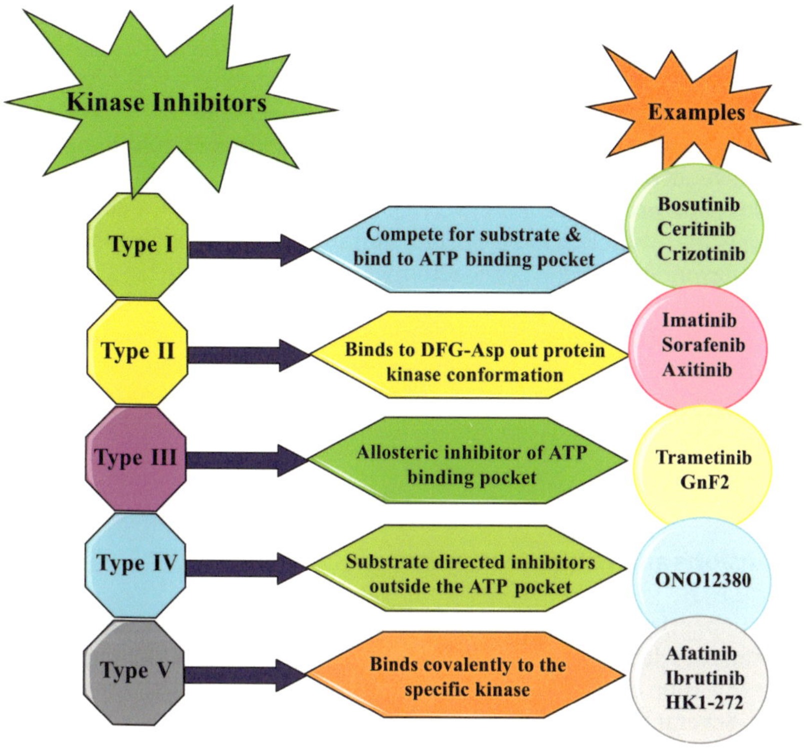

Figure 2.
Inhibitory patterns of different kinase inhibitors.

From a clinical point of view, it has been observed that kinase target anticancer therapies have more success rate than the other cancer therapies. But it is also evident in the past few years EGFR/VEGF-targeting molecules have given unsatisfactory results [64, 65]. Instead, success stories have been seen with molecules targeting kinase B, phosphatidylinositol kinase delta and gamma, kinase I, tyrosine kinase, nerve growth receptors Wee 1-like kinases in Phase 1 clinical trials. The latest explored targets Aurora kinases have led to the development of two inhibitors palbociclib and ribociclib which have passed phase III clinical trials [66]. The modern developments on kinases are following the precision therapy that has been based upon the genomic data. The detailed genetic studies on tumors and drivers involved in the generation of tumors have resulted in tremendous advantages for patients who need effective therapy.

3. Investigations on kinase inhibitory potentials of natural products

The continuous research is in progress for several years to design synthetic and natural chemotherapeutic agents against cancer with selective cytotoxic efficacy and minimum toxicity [67–70]. The contribution of molecules from natural sources in kinase-mediated anticancer research cannot be ignored. The kinase modulating properties of natural molecules has brought a new paradigm in the screening of kinase inhibitors. Toward this direction, small molecules like polyphenols have revealed tremendous potentials to bind with kinases like tyrosine kinase followed by alteration of phosphorylation leading to modulation of multi-signaling mechanisms. The explored natural compounds in this direction are curcumins, resveratrol, quercetin, cyrysitin, myricetin, luteolin, apigenin, anthocyanin, genistein, epigallocatechin gallate, fisetin, astaxanthin, and tetrahydrocurcumins and many more. Polyphenols such as resveratrol [71], quercetin [72], curcumin [73] and tea extracts [74] have revealed promising EGFR inhibition [75]. Curcumin and chrysin have receptor RON blocker activity in tumor cells [76, 77]. Natural products have also shown Abl, JAK-2, c-Met, c-SRC, and serine kinase inhibitory potentials [78–80]. Resveratrol also has modulatory effects on the expression of Akt in breast, uterine, skin, and prostate cancers [81, 82]. It binds to the ATP site competitively as well as reversibly. Myricetin has reported inhibition of cell proliferation by binding to Akt. Beyond these significant activities, several reports in the literature are available evidencing the inhibitory and modulatory effects of natural products on mTOR, CDK, Aurora kinases, B-raf kinases, PI3K [83–85], etc. Many natural molecules bind directly to the oncogenic kinases and alter the cell signaling involved in tumor progression by modifying the phosphorylation process. Several other classes of natural compounds are under investigation for their kinase-modulating activities.

4. Conclusions and future perspectives

The therapeutic implication of protein kinases against a variety of cancers is well known from past decades. Also, it is well established that deregulation, mutations, and overexpression of these kinases are important triggers for the development of cancers. Several kinase inhibitors are already reported who prevent cancer by modulating the protein kinases by following different mechanisms and several inhibitors are under investigation. Despite tremendous advancements in kinase drug development, still, a large number of kinases are unexplored. It is also worth notable that most of the available kinase inhibitors work through binding to ATP sites. A great challenge in clinical implication of kinase inhibitors is the development of drug resistance of cancer stem cells. It develops due to the loss of activity of some important kinases. Therefore, strategies to overcome this resistance are the requirement of the hour. In the therapeutics of cancer, the kinase inhibitors have been proven to be well tolerated as compared to the traditional therapies.

Abbreviations

ABL	Abelson murine leukemia viral oncogene
Abl	Abelson murine leukemia
Akt	protein kinase B
ALK	anaplastic lymphoma kinase
BRAF	proto-oncogene
BTK	Bruton agammaglobulinemia tyrosine kinase
CDK	cyclin-dependent kinase
c-Met	c-MET proto-oncogene
c-SRC	proto-oncogene tyrosine-protein kinase
CTK	cytoplasmic tyrosine kinase
EGFR	epidermal growth factor receptor
ERBB2	V-Erb-B2 avian erythroblastic leukemia viral oncogene homolog
FGFRs	fibroblast growth factor receptors
HER-2	human epidermal growth factorreceptor-2
JAK2	Janus kinase 2
MAPK	mitogen-activated protein kinases
MEK	MEK kinase gene

PDGFRs	platelet-derived growth factor receptors
PI3K	phosphatidylinositol-3-kinase
PI3KCA	phosphatidylinositol-4,5-bisphosphate 3-kinase
RTK	receptor tyrosine kinase
VEGFR-2	vascular endothelial growth factor receptor 2

Author details

Rohit Bhatia[1] and Rajesh K. Singh[2]*

1 Department of Pharmaceutical Chemistry, ISF College of Pharmacy, Moga, Punjab, India

2 Department of Pharmaceutical Chemistry, Shivalik College of Pharmacy, Nangal, Punjab, India

*Address all correspondence to: rksingh244@gmail.com

References

[1] Bhatia R, Rawal RK. Coumarin hybrids: Promising scaffolds in the treatment of breast cancer. Mini Reviews in Medicinal Chemistry. 2019;**19**(17):1443-1458

[2] Nagai H, Kim YH. Cancer prevention from the perspective of global cancer burden patterns. Journal of Thoracic Disease. 2017;**9**(3):448-451

[3] Bhullar KS, Lagarón NO, McGowan EM, et al. Kinase-targeted cancer therapies: Progress, challenges and future directions. Molecular Cancer. 2018;**17**:48

[4] Berndt N, Karim RM, Schönbrunn E. Advances of small molecule targeting of kinases. Current Opinion in Chemical Biology. 2017;**39**:126-132

[5] Cohen P, Cross D, Jänne PA. Kinase drug discovery 20 years after imatinib: Progress and future directions. Nature Reviews. Drug Discovery. 2021;**20**: 551-569

[6] Pottier C, Fresnais M, Gilon M, Jérusalem G, Longuespée R, Sounni NE. Tyrosine kinase inhibitors in cancer: Breakthrough and challenges of targeted therapy. Cancers. 2020;**12**(3):731

[7] Yu JS, Cui W. Proliferation, survival and metabolism: The role of PI3K/AKT/mTOR signalling in pluripotency and cell fate determination. Development. 2016;**143**:3050-3060

[8] Ardito F, Giuliani M, Perrone D, Troiano G, Lo ML. The crucial role of protein phosphorylation in cell signaling and its use as targeted therapy (review). International Journal of Molecular Medicine. 2017;**40**(2):271-280

[9] Lemmon MA, Schlessinger J. Cell signaling by receptor tyrosine kinases. Cell. 2010;**141**:1117-1134

[10] Cooke M, Magimaidas A, Casado-Medrano V, Kazanietz MG. Protein kinase C in cancer: The top five unanswered questions. Molecular Carcinogenesis. 2017;**56**:1531-1542

[11] Bononi A, Agnoletto C, De Marchi E, et al. Protein kinases and phosphatases in the control of cell fate. Enzyme Research. 2011;**2011**:329098

[12] Kannaiyan R, Mahadevan D. A comprehensive review of protein kinase inhibitors for cancer therapy. Expert Review of Anticancer Therapy. 2018;**18**(12):1249-1270

[13] Alkharsah KR. VEGF upregulation in viral infections and its possible therapeutic implications. International Journal of Molecular Sciences. 2018;**19**(6):1642

[14] Soroceanu L, Akhavan A, Cobbs CS. Platelet-derived growth factor-alpha receptor activation is required for human cytomegalovirus infection. Nature. 2008;**455**(7211):391-395

[15] Nukaga S, Yasuda H, Tsuchihara K, Hamamoto J, Masuzawa K, Kawada I, et al. Amplification of egfr wild-type alleles in non-small cell lung cancer cells confers acquired resistance to mutation-selective egfr tyrosine kinase inhibitors. Cancer Research. 2017;**77**:2078-2089

[16] Khan SA, Zeng Z, Shia J, Paty PB. Egfr gene amplification and kras mutation predict response to combination targeted therapy in metastatic colorectal cancer. Pathology Oncology Research. 2017;**23**:673-677

[17] Zhou C, Zhu L, Ji J, Ding F, Wang C, Cai Q, et al. Egfr high expression, but not kras status, predicts sensitivity of pancreatic cancer cells to nimotuzumab treatment in vivo. Current Cancer Drug Targets. 2017;**17**:89-97

[18] Morey AL, Brown B, Farshid G, Fox SB, Francis GD, McCue G, et al. Determining her2 (erbb2) amplification status in women with breast cancer: Final results from the australian in situ hybridisation program. Pathology. 2016;**48**:535-542

[19] Wang YK, Yang BF, Yun T, Zhu CY, Li CY, Jiang B, et al. Methods and significance of the combined detection of her2 gene amplification and chemosensitivity in gastric cancer. Cancer Biomarkers. 2017;**21**:439-447

[20] Xu CW, Wang WX, Wu MJ, Zhu YC, Zhuang W, Lin G, et al. Comparison of the c-met gene amplification between primary tumor and metastatic lymph nodes in non-small cell lung cancer. Thoracic Cancer. 2017;**8**:417-422

[21] Blanke CD, Demetri GD, von Mehren M, Heinrich MC, Eisenberg B, Fletcher JA, et al. Long-term results from a randomized phase II trial of standard versus higher-dose imatinib mesylate for patients with unresectable or metastatic gastrointestinal stromal tumors expressing KIT. Journal of Clinical Oncology. 2008;**26**:620-625

[22] Cohen P. Protein kinases—The major drug targets of the twenty-first century? Nature Reviews. Drug Discovery. 2002;**1**:309-315

[23] Wedam S, Fashoyin-Aje L, Bloomquist E, Tang S, Sridhara R, Goldberg KB, et al. FDA approval summary: Palbociclib for male patients with metastatic breast cancer. Clinical Cancer Research. 2020;**26**(6):1208-1212

[24] Nair A, Reece K, Donoghue MB, Yuan WV, Rodriguez L, Keegan P, et al. FDA supplemental approval summary: Lenvatinib for the treatment of unresectable hepatocellular carcinoma. The Oncologist. 2021;**26**(3):e484-e491

[25] https://www.fda.gov/drugs/resources-information-approved-drugs/fda-approves-osimertinib-first-line-treatment-metastatic-nsclc-most-common-egfr-mutations [Accessed: 4 September 2021]

[26] Greig SL. Osimertinib: First global approval. Drugs. 2016;**76**(2):263-273

[27] Fala LP. Necitumumab: An IgG1 monoclonal antibody, FDA approved for advanced squamous non-small-cell lung cancer. American Health & Drug Benefits. 2016;**9**(Spec Feature):119-122

[28] Larkins E, Blumenthal GM, Chen H, He K, Agarwal R, Gieser G, et al. FDA approval: Alectinib for the treatment of metastatic, ALK-positive non-small cell lung cancer following crizotinib. Clinical Cancer Research. 2016;**22**(21):5171-5176

[29] Shirley M. Olaratumab: First global approval. Drugs. 2017;**77**(1):107-112

[30] Shah A, Bloomquist E, Tang S, Fu W, Bi Y, Liu Q, et al. FDA approval: Ribociclib for the treatment of postmenopausal women with hormone receptor-positive, HER2-negative advanced or metastatic breast cancer. Clinical Cancer Research. 2018;**24**(13):2999-3004

[31] https://www.fda.gov/drugs/resources-information-approved-drugs/brigatinib [Accessed: 4 September 2021]

[32] Kumar A, Bhatia R, Chawla P, Anghore D, Saini V, Rawal RK. Copanlisib: Novel PI3K inhibitor for the treatment of lymphoma. Anti-Cancer Agents in Medicinal Chemistry. 2020;**20**(10):1158-1172

[33] Voli L, Mamyrbékova J, Bazureau J. Abemaciclib, a recent novel FDA-Approved small molecule inhibiting cyclin-dependant kinase 4/6 for the treatment of metastatic breast cancer: A mini-review. Open Journal of Medicinal Chemistry. 2020;**10**:128-138

[34] https://www.cancer.gov/news-events/cancer-currents-blog/2017/acalabrutinib-fda-mantle-cell-lymphoma [Accessed: 4 September 2021]

[35] Shirley M. Encorafenib and binimetinib: First global approvals. Drugs. 2018;**78**(12):1277-1284

[36] Kopetz S, Grothey A, Yaeger R, Van Cutsem E, Desai J, Yoshino T, et al. Encorafenib, binimetinib, and cetuximab in *BRAF* V600E-mutated colorectal cancer. The New England Journal of Medicine. 2019;**381**(17): 1632-1643

[37] Rodrigues DA, Sagrillo FS, Fraga CAM. Duvelisib: A 2018 novel FDA-approved small molecule inhibiting phosphoinositide 3-kinases. Pharmaceuticals. 2019;**12**(2):69

[38] Shirley M. Dacomitinib: First global approval. Drugs. 2018;**78**(18):1947-1953

[39] Solomon BJ, Besse B, Bauer TM, Felip E, Soo RA, Camidge DR, et al. Lorlatinib in patients with ALK-positive non-small-cell lung cancer: Results from a global phase 2 study. The Lancet Oncology. 2018;**19**(12):1654-1667

[40] Perl AE, Martinelli G, Cortes JE, Neubauer A, Berman E, Paolini S, et al. Gilteritinib or chemotherapy for relapsed or refractory *FLT3*-mutated AML. The New England Journal of Medicine. 2019;**381**(18):1728-1740

[41] Montazeri K, Bellmunt J. Erdafitinib for the treatment of metastatic bladder cancer. Expert Review of Clinical Pharmacology. 2020;**13**(1):1-6

[42] Tayyar Y, Idris A, Vidimce J, Ferreira DA, McMillan NA. Alpelisib and radiotherapy treatment enhances Alisertib-mediated cervical cancer tumor killing. American Journal of Cancer Research. 2021;**11**(6):3240-3251

[43] Benner B, Good L, Quiroga D, et al. Pexidartinib, a novel small molecule CSF-1R inhibitor in use for tenosynovial giant cell tumor: A systematic review of pre-clinical and clinical development. Drug Design, Development and Therapy. 2020;**14**:1693-1704

[44] Sartore-Bianchi A, Pizzutilo EG, Marrapese G, Tosi F, Cerea G, Siena S. Entrectinib for the treatment of metastatic NSCLC: Safety and efficacy. Expert Review of Anticancer Therapy. 2020;**20**(5):333-341

[45] Trotman J, Opat S, Gottlieb D, Simpson D, Marlton P, Cull G, et al. Zanubrutinib for the treatment of patients with Waldenström macroglobulinemia: 3 years of follow-up. Blood. 2020;**136**(18): 2027-2037

[46] Heinrich MC, Jones RL, von Mehren M, Schöffski P, Serrano C, Kang YK, et al. Avapritinib in advanced PDGFRA D842V-mutant gastrointestinal stromal tumour (NAVIGATOR): A multicentre, open-label, phase 1 trial. The Lancet Oncology. 2020;**21**:7935-7946

[47] Gross AM, Wolters PL, Dombi E, Baldwin A, Whitcomb P, Fisher MJ, et al. Selumetinib in children with inoperable plexiform neurofibromas. The New England Journal of Medicine. 2020;**382**:1430-1442

[48] Murth RK, Loi S, Okines A, Paplomata E, Hamilton E, Hurvitz SA, et al. Tucatinib, trastuzumab, and capecitabine for HER2-positive metastatic breast cancer. The New England Journal of Medicine. 2020;**382**:597-609

[49] Abou-Alfa GK, Sahai V, Hollebecque A, Vaccaro G, Melisi D, Al-Rajabi R, et al. Pemigatinib for previously treated, locally advanced or metastatic cholangiocarcinoma:

A multicentre, open-label, phase 2 study. The Lancet Oncology. 2020;**21**:671-684

[50] Wolf J, Seto T, Han JY, Reguart N, Garon EB, Groen HJM, et al. Capmatinibin MET exon 14-mutated or MET-amplified non-small-cell lung cancer. The New England Journal of Medicine. 2020;**383**:944-957

[51] Wirth LJ, Sherman E, Robinson B, Solomon B, Kang H, Lorch J, et al. Efficacy of selpercatinib in RET-altered thyroid cancers. The New England Journal of Medicine. 2020;**383**:825-835

[52] Blay JY, Serrano C, Heinrich MC, Zalcberg J, Bauer S, Gelderblom H, et al. Ripretinib in patients with advanced gastrointestinal stromal tumours (INVICTUS): A double-blind, randomised, placebo controlled, phase 3 trial. The Lancet Oncology. 2020;**21**: 923-934

[53] Hu M, Subbiah V, Wirth LJ, Schuler M, Mansfield AS, Brose MS, et al. Results from the registrational phase I/II ARROW trial of pralsetinib (BLU-667) in patients (pts) with advanced RET mutation positive medullary thyroid cancer (RET + MTC). ESMO Virtual Congress. 2020;**31**:S1084

[54] Rugo HS, Im SA, Cardoso F, Cortés J, Curigliano G, Musolino A, et al. Efficacy of margetuximab vs trastuzumab in patients with pretreated ERBB2-positive advanced breast cancer: A phase 3 randomized clinical trial. JAMA Oncology. 2021;7(4):573-584

[55] Tam CS, Opat S, Simpson D, Cull G, Munoz J, Phillips TJ, et al. Zanubrutinib for the treatment of relapsed or refractory mantle cell lymphoma. Blood Advances. 2021;**5**(12):2577-2585

[56] Huynh H, Lee LY, Goh KY, et al. Infigratinib mediates vascular normalization, impairs metastasis, and improves chemotherapy in hepatocellular carcinoma. Hepatology. 2019;**69**(3):943-958

[57] Tanaka H, Taima K, Makiguchi T, Nakagawa J, Niioka T, Tasaka S. Activity and bioavailability of tepotinib for leptomeningeal metastasis of NSCLC with MET exon 14 skipping mutation. Cancer Communications. 2021;**41**(1): 83-87

[58] https://www.fda.gov/drugs/resources-information-approved-drugs/fda-approves-tivozanib-relapsed-or-refractory-advanced-renal-cell-carcinoma [Accessed: 4 September 2021]

[59] Jonker DJ, O'Callaghan CJ, Karapetis CS, Zalcberg JR, Tu D, Au H-J, et al. Cetuximab for the treatment of colorectal cancer. The New England Journal of Medicine. 2007;**357**: 2040-2048

[60] Hudis CA. Trastuzumab—Mechanism of action and use in clinical practice. The New England Journal of Medicine. 2007;**357**:39-51

[61] Dar AC, Shokat KM. The evolution of protein kinase inhibitors from antagonists to agonists of cellular signaling. Annual Review of Biochemistry. 2011;**80**:769-795

[62] Roskoski R. Classification of small molecule protein kinase inhibitors based upon the structures of their drug-enzyme complexes. Pharmacological Research. 2016;**103**:26-48

[63] Zuccotto F, Ardini E, Casale E, Angiolini M. Through the "gatekeeper door": Exploiting the active kinase conformation. Journal of Medicinal Chemistry. 2009;**53**:2681-2694

[64] Takeda M, Nakagawa K. Toxicity profile of epidermal growth factor receptor tyrosine kinase inhibitors in

patients with epidermal growth factor receptor gene mutation-positive lung cancer. Molecular and Clinical Oncology. 2017;**6**:3-6

[65] Yr L, Zhu W, Jl Z, Jq H, Zhao YZ, Zhang W, et al. The evaluation of efficacy and safety of sunitinib on EGFR-TKI pretreated advanced non-small cell lung cancer patients in China. The Clinical Respiratory Journal. 2014;**8**:206-212

[66] Knapp S, Sundström M. Recently targeted kinases and their inhibitors—The path to clinical trials. Current Opinion in Pharmacology. 2014;**17**:58-63

[67] Kumar S, Sharma B, Bhardwaj TR, Singh RK. Design, synthesis and studies on novel polymeric prodrugs of erlotinib for colon drug delivery. Anti-Cancer Agents in Medicinal Chemistry. 2021;**21**(3):383-392

[68] Singh RK, Prasad DN, Bhardwaj TR. Synthesis, in vitro/in vivo evaluation and in silico physicochemical study of prodrug approach for brain targeting of alkylating agent. Medicinal Chemistry Research. 2013;**22**:5324-5336

[69] Singh RK, Kumar S, Prasad DN, Bhardwaj TR. Therapeutic journey of nitrogen mustard as alkylating anticancer agents: Historic to future perspectives. European Journal of Medicinal Chemistry. 2018;**151**:401-433

[70] Singh RK, Kumar S, Prasad DN, Bhardwaj TR. Reversible redox system based drug design for targeting alkylating agent across brain. Medicinal Chemistry Research. 2014;**23**(5): 2405-2416

[71] Jeong KJ, Cho KH, Panupinthu N, Kim H, Kang J, Park CG, et al. EGFR mediates LPA-induced proteolytic enzyme expression and ovarian cancer invasion: Inhibition by resveratrol. Molecular Oncology. 2013;**7**:121-129

[72] Huang C-Y, Chan C-Y, Chou I-T, Lien C-H, Hung H-C, Lee M-F. Quercetin induces growth arrest through activation of FOXO1 transcription factor in EGFR-overexpressing oral cancer cells. The Journal of Nutritional Biochemistry. 2013;**24**:1596-1603

[73] Sun X-D, Liu X-E, Huang D-S. Curcumin induces apoptosis of triple-negative breast cancer cells by inhibition of EGFR expression. Molecular Medicine Reports. 2012;**6**:1267-1270

[74] Masuda M, Wakasaki T, Toh S, Shimizu M, Adachi S. Chemoprevention of head and neck cancer by green tea extract: EGCG—The role of EGFR signaling and "lipid raft". Journal of Oncology. 2011;**2011**:540148

[75] Nicholson R, Gee J, Harper M. EGFR and cancer prognosis. European Journal of Cancer. 2001;**37**:9-15

[76] Sakurai R, Villarreal P, Husain S, Liu J, Sakurai T, Tou E, et al. Curcumin protects the developing lung against long-term hyperoxic injury. American Journal of Physiology—Lung Cellular and Molecular Physiology. 2013;**305**: L301-L311

[77] Narasimhan M, Ammanamanchi S. Curcumin blocks RON tyrosine kinase-mediated invasion of breast carcinoma cells. Cancer Research. 2008;**68**: 5185-5192

[78] Greuber EK, Smith-Pearson P, Wang J, Pendergast AM. Role of ABL family kinases in cancer: From leukaemia to solid tumours. Nature Reviews. Cancer. 2013;**13**:559-571

[79] Byun S, Lee KW, Jung SK, Lee EJ, Hwang MK, Lim SH, et al. Luteolin inhibits protein kinase Cε and c-Src activities and UVB induced skin cancer. Cancer Research. 2010;**70**:2415-2423

[80] Wolanin K, Magalska A, Mosieniak G, Klinger R, Mckenna S, Vejda S, et al. Curcumin affects components of the chromosomal passenger complex and induces mitotic catastrophe in apoptosis-resistant Bcr-Abl expressing cells. Molecular Cancer Research. 2006;**4**:457-469

[81] Jiang H, Shang X, Wu H, Gautam SC, Al-Holou S, Li C, et al. Resveratrol downregulates PI3K/Akt/mTOR signaling pathways in human U251 glioma cells. Journal of Experimental Therapeutics & Oncology. 2009;**8**:25

[82] Fröjdö S, Cozzone D, Vidal H, Pirola L. Resveratrol is a class IA phosphoinositide 3-kinase inhibitor. The Biochemical Journal. 2007;**406**:511-518

[83] Park D, Jeong H, Lee MN, Koh A, Kwon O, Yang YR, et al. Resveratrol induces autophagy by directly inhibiting mTOR through ATP competition. Scientific Reports. 2016;**6**:21772

[84] Kumamoto T, Fujii M, Hou D-X. Akt is a direct target for myricetin to inhibit cell transformation. Molecular and Cellular Biochemistry. 2009;**332**:33-41

[85] Weir NM, Selvendiran K, Kutala VK, Tong L, Vishwanath S, Rajaram M, et al. Curcumin induces G2/M arrest and apoptosis in cisplatin-resistant human ovarian cancer cells by modulating Akt and p38 MAPK. Cancer Biology and Therapy. 2007;**6**:178-184

Chapter 2

Protein Kinase Inhibitors - Selectivity or Toxicity?

Moran Grossman and Elaine Adler

Abstract

Protein kinases are attractive therapeutic targets for various indications including cancer, cardiovascular, neurodegenerative and autoimmune diseases. This is due to the fact that they play key roles in the regulation of cell cycle, metabolism, cell adhesion, angiogenesis, regeneration and degeneration. Protein kinase families share a common catalytic core and hence usually display clear sequence and structural similarity. These sequence and structural similarities can lead to a lack of selectivity and off-target toxicity of drug candidates. The lack of selectivity can be beneficial but can also cause adverse toxicities which result in the discontinuation of promising drug candidates. The chapter reviews the challenges and common toxicities of protein kinase inhibitors and the latest advances in in-vitro and in-silico assays to screen for selectivity. The various methods for quantifying selectivity of kinase inhibitors and future directions including emerging more selective and safer kinase inhibitors have also been discussed.

Keywords: Selectivity, Kinase inhibitors, Toxicity

1. Introduction

Protein kinases belong to a huge family of more than 500 enzymes that phosphorylate proteins in response to an external stimulus, via transfer of the γ-phosphate group from ATP to serine, threonine, or tyrosine residues on the target protein [1]. By doing so they regulate the function of many proteins, and mediate and influence a variety of cellular processes including proliferation, metabolism, adhesion, angiogenesis, regeneration and degeneration [2]. Since most protein kinases are involved in pivotal biological reactions, it is not surprising that dysregulation of the activities of kinases is the hallmark of many pathological conditions such as cancer [3], autoimmunity [4], inflammation [5], and neurological disorders [6]. In particular, genetic alteration in various protein kinases is associated with their over-expression and disease pathology, but also with drug response and resistance. Accordingly, more than 250 kinase inhibitors (KIs) are currently undergoing clinical trials and more than 50 have been approved for use by the Food and Drug Administration (FDA) [7]. Even though most therapeutic agents are mainly for oncologic indications such as imatinib (first small molecule KI approved for chemotherapy in 2001), gefitinib, sorafinib, erlotinib, dasatinib and crizotinib, there are also emerging KIs for other indications such as rheumatoid arthritis (RA), inflammatory bowel disease, alopecia areata, psoriasis, idiopathic pulmonary fibrosis, organ rejection prophylaxis, glaucoma and neurodegenerative diseases such as Alzheimer disease [8]. In fact, KIs have become one of the most prevalent druggable

IntechOpen

targets with an estimated one-third of drug discovery programs aimed at developing KIs. Kinase inhibitors have transformed the treatment of many cancers and are showing the same promise for other indications. However, their development has been challenging due to severe toxicities observed in preclinical studies and clinical trials [9, 10].

Most of the approved KIs are small molecules, which may be classified into six main groups according to their binding site on the enzyme [11, 12]: KIs which bind to the ATP pocket in the active conformation of a kinase are classified as Type I; KIs that bind adjacent to the ATP pocket (adenine binding residues) of the unphosphorylated inactive conformation of kinases are classified as Type II; non-ATP competitive inhibitors that bind within the cleft between the small and large lobes close to the ATP binding pocket are classified as Type III; allosteric inhibitors that bind away from the ATP cleft are classified as Type IV; agents that span two distinct regions of the protein kinase domain are classified type V inhibitors; and agents that form covalent bonds with their target enzyme are classified type VI inhibitors [7].

These different binding modes not only influence the potency and mechanism of action of these inhibitors, but may also affect their selectivity and consequently their safety profile. Since type I inhibitors bind to the well-conserved ATP binding site shared by most protein kinases, these inhibitors are often less selective, and interact with multiple members of the protein kinase family. For example, most of the ATP-competitive inhibitors such as imatinib, nilotinib, dasatinib, bosutinib, and ponatinib that successfully target the oncoprotein kinase ABL1, exhibit notable off-target activities on kinases such as c-KIT, CSF1R, and PDGFRA/B [8] **Figure 1** shows an

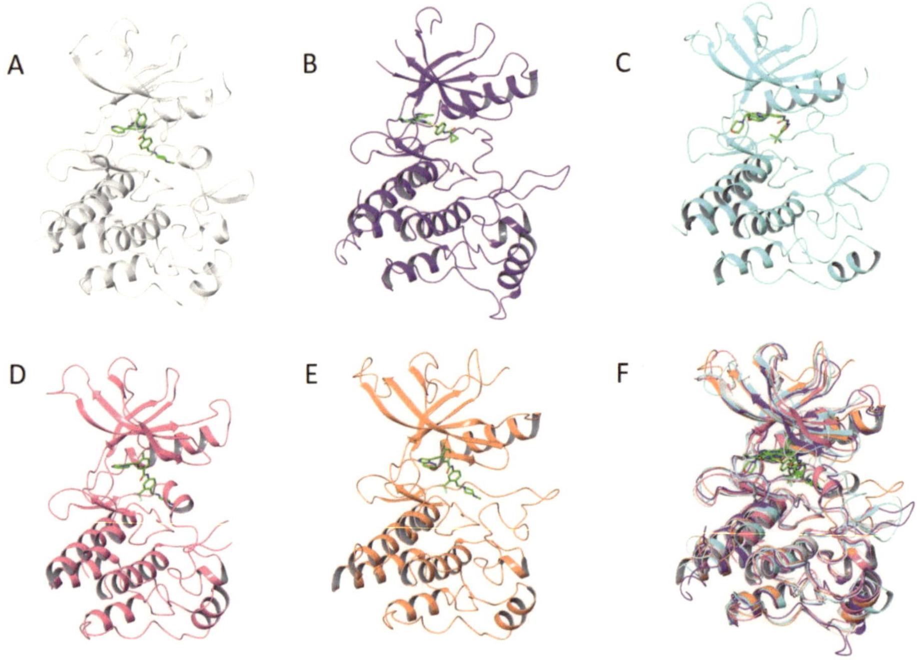

Figure 1.
Crystal structures of representative kinases complexed with small molecule inhibitors at the conserved ATP active site. A) Human Abl kinase domain in complex with imatinib. PDB ID: 2HYY. B) DDR1 bound to VX-680. PDB ID: 6BRJ. C) Crystal structure of the FLT3 kinase domain bound to the inhibitor quizartinib, PDB ID: 4XUF. D) The ROR1 Pseudokinase Domain Bound To Ponatinib. PDB ID: 6TU9. E) FGFR4 in complex with Ponatinib. PDB: 4UXQ. F) overlay of the five crystal structures (A-E) showing the high structural homology between the different kinases. The small molecule inhibitors are shown in green sticks. Images were drawn using the maestro software [13].

overlay of the crystal structures of five representative kinases from different families with their respective small molecule inhibitors bound to the ATP active site, demonstrating why type I inhibitors usually have low selectivity. This cross reactivity is associated with toxicities in the clinic and often leads to discontinuation of promising drug candidates during development as will be described in this chapter. Type II KIs demonstrate improved selectivity profiles compared with type I inhibitors because they bind adjacent to the ATP binding pocket in the inactive kinase conformational state, a site which is less conserved within the kinome [14]. Type III-VI inhibitors, which are non-ATP competitive inhibitors that often do not bind to conserved residues, offer greater selectivity and reduced toxicity compared to other types of KIs as they are likely to have less off-target effects [15–17]. In addition, the toxicity profiles of KIs depend on which kinase was targeted, the affinity of the inhibitor for the particular kinase and on the role that this kinase plays in intracellular signaling and overall cell function.

Off-target activity of KIs are not necessarily limited to kinases. Non-kinase off-targets of KIs often remain undiscovered, and may lead to misinterpretation of the cause of toxicity [18]. That is, KIs may also bind to other enzymes, ion channels and/or receptors and thus performing a full binding profile is important to understand all potential targets as well as subsequently assessing off-target activity. However, off-target activity is not always a cause for concern for therapeutic agents as the off-target activity may have positive therapeutic outcomes. Multi-targeted KIs may target a pathway at different points e.g. upstream and downstream and thus multi-targeted KIs may have improved efficacy compared to more selective inhibitors. Additionally, KIs with off-target activity in different pathways may be beneficial for targeting different indications [19, 20].

In addition to small molecule inhibitors, there are also several monoclonal antibodies (mAbs) that specifically and selectively target and block the extracellular domain of receptor tyrosine kinases such as epidermal growth factor receptor (EGFR, HER1, ErbB-1), and human epidermal growth factor receptor 2 (HER2, ErbB-2) [21]. By targeting the extracellular part of the receptor tyrosine kinase, the mAb is able to block the binding of the natural ligand, avoid receptor conformational rearrangement essential to the activation of the kinase and thus the activation of the downstream signaling pathways. Even though mAbs therapies are often considered as very specific and safer therapeutic agents, anti-EGFR antibodies, such as cetuximab and panitumumab, have been associated with severe skin, renal, and gastrointestinal toxicities as they block essential cellular signaling pathways [22, 23]. In addition, the development of chemoresistance in a large portion of patients due to the ability of cells to re-activate pro-angiogenic factors via alternate pathways (i.e. increasing VEGF production), also hampered the success of these drugs in the clinic [24].

This chapter will review the challenges of developing safe protein KIs, the latest advances in assays to screen for selectivity and future directions.

2. Common toxicities with kinase inhibitors

Adverse effects from KIs may be classified into on- and off-target toxicities. "On-target" toxicity results when the inhibition of the targeted kinase is responsible for both the intended pharmacodynamic effect and the unintended toxicity. On the contrary, "off-target" toxicity is the result of low selectivity and inhibition of kinases for which the drug was not intended.

KIs are associated with undesirable adverse reactions that impact on quality of life and compliance of patients, even though less than traditional chemotherapy.

These effects include cardiovascular toxicity, hepatotoxicity, hematotoxicity, dermatological and ocular toxicities, gastro-intestinal symptoms, hyperphosphatemia and tissue mineralization [25]. For example, EGFR-Tyrosine KIs (TKIs) are typically associated skin rash, diarrhea, hepatotoxicity, stomatitis, interstitial lung disease and ocular toxicity, but these effects are usually mild in most cases [26]. In this chapter we decided to focus on the mechanism of three major toxicities: cardiovascular toxicity, hepatotoxicity and hematotoxicity. This decision was not based on the incidence of the side effects but rather the impact of these particular side effects on patients. These side effects have a great impact on patients due to the effects on their well-being and compliance to treatment. In addition, these particular side effects are a major cause for discontinuing the development of many molecules. Therefore, improving the selectivity of compounds in a manner that will not interfere with or avoid the mechanisms outlined below is important.

2.1 Cardiovascular toxicity

Many protein kinases are critical for normal function of cardiomyocytes and/or the vasculature, and thus their inhibition results in "on-target" cardiotoxicity due to the overlap in the targeted pathway for cancer progression and the pathway for regulation of cardiac function [27]. Protein kinase signaling plays a significant role in cardiac hypertrophy (increase in cell size) under physiological conditions in response to an increased workload, such as exercise or pregnancy, but the relative importance of individual kinases is not clear. Microarray analysis of protein kinase mRNA expression in dozens of non-failing human heart biopsies detected 402 protein kinase mRNAs that are constantly expressed under normal, non-pathologic conditions [28]. Therefore, it is not surprising that many KIs have a cardiovascular (CV) toxicity warning and precautions in their US prescribing information. The adverse cardiac events listed in the US prescribing information for cancer patients following treatment with KIs include: QT prolongation, hypertension, left ventricular dysfunction (LVD), congestive heart failure (CHF), acute coronary syndromes (ACS), and myocardial infarction (MI) [27]. For example, targeting VEGF is associated with hypertension, and targeting human epidermal growth factor receptor 2 (HER2), VEGFR, and/or Bcr-Abl is often accompanied with LVD and CHF [29, 30]. The consequence cardiac toxicity among new KIs due to "on-target" activities and lack of selectivity, limits development of new drugs even when targeting life-threatening therapeutic indications such as cancer.

Not all KIs, however, are prone to cardiotoxicity. More selective KIs targeting the Janus kinase (JAK) family, such as tofacitinib targeting Janus kinase (JAK) 1/3 for the treatment of RA, psoriatic arthritis, ulcerative colitis, and the selective JAK2 inhibitor, fedratinib, are not associated with cardiotoxicity (see **Table 1**). Similarly, inhibitors of mammalian target of rapamycin (mTOR) such as sirolimus, temsirolimus and everolimus developed for different malignancies are also not accompanied with cardiotoxicity (see **Table 1**, US prescribing information for sirolimus, temsirolimus and everolimus) despite the role of mTOR signaling in cardiac physiology [31]. These examples demonstrate that cardiotoxicity may be overcome by increasing selectivity.

2.2 Hepatotoxicity

Hepatotoxicity has been reported for several TKIs and it is estimated to affect approximately 5% of patients [32]. The clinical effects have ranged from mild elevation in transaminases to progressive irreversible cirrhosis, which has resulted in death, and are dependent on the specific interaction between the drugs and the

Drug	Year of approval	primary target	Indication	Most common adverse reactions and warnings (as mentions in the US prescribing information)
BCR-Abl inhibitors				
Bosutinib	2012	BCR-Abl	Chronic myelogenous leukemias	Diarrhea, nausea, thrombocytopenia, rash, increased alanine aminotransferase, abdominal pain, increased aspartate aminotransferase, thrombocytopenia, vomiting, anemia, fatigue, pyrexia, cough, headache, alanine aminotransferase, and edema
Dasatinib	2006	BCR-Abl, SRC kinase	Chronic myelogenous leukemias	Myelosuppression (thrombocytopenia, neutropenia, and anemia may occur), fluid retention events, diarrhea, headache, skin rash, hemorrhage, dyspnea, fatigue, nausea, and musculoskeletal pain
Imatinib	2001	BCR-Abl	Philadelphia chromosome-positive CML or ALL, aggressive systemic mastocytosis, chronic eosinophilic leukemias, dermatofibrosarcoma protuberans, hypereosinophilic syndrome, gastrointestinal stromal tumors, myelodysplastic/ myeloproliferative disease	Cytopenias, particularly anemia, neutropenia, and thrombocytopenia, hepatotoxicity, heart failure and left ventricular dysfunction, edema, nausea, vomiting, muscle cramps, musculoskeletal pain, diarrhea, rash, fatigue and abdominal pain
EGFR and VEGFR inhibitors				
Cetuximab	2004	EGFR	Head and neck cancer and colorectal cancer	Fatal infusion reactions and Cardiopulmonary arrest. Cutaneous adverse reactions (including rash, pruritus, and nail changes), headache, diarrhea, and infection
Panitumumab	2006	EGFR	Colorectal Cancer	Skin toxicities (i.e., erythema, dermatitis acneiform, pruritus, exfoliation, rash, and fissures), paronychia, hypomagnesemia, fatigue, abdominal pain, nausea, diarrhea, and constipation
Erlotinib	2004	EGFR	NSCLC, pancreatic cancers	NSCLC: rash, diarrhea, anorexia, fatigue, dyspnea, cough, nausea, infection and vomiting. Pancreatic cancer: fatigue, rash, nausea, anorexia, diarrhea, abdominal pain, vomiting, weight decrease, infection, edema, pyrexia, constipation, bone pain, dyspnea, stomatitis and myalgia.
Gefitinib	2015	EGFR	NSCLC	Skin reactions and diarrhea, interstitial lung disease and Hepatotoxicity

Drug	Year of approval	primary target	Indication	Most common adverse reactions and warnings (as mentions in the US prescribing information)
Lapatinib	2007	HER2 and EGFR	HER2-positive breast cancers	Hepatotoxicity, diarrhea, palmar-plantar erythrodysesthesia, nausea, rash, vomiting, and fatigue. May prolong the QT interval in some patients or decreases in left ventricular ejection fraction,
Pazopanib	2009	VEGFR	Advanced renal cell carcinoma, advanced soft tissue sarcoma	Hepatotoxicity Advanced renal cell carcinoma: diarrhea, hypertension, hair color changes (depigmentation), nausea, anorexia, and vomiting. Advanced soft tissue sarcoma: fatigue, diarrhea, nausea, decreased weight, hypertension, decreased appetite, vomiting, tumor pain, hair color changes, musculoskeletal pain, headache, dysgeusia, dyspnea and skin hypopigmentation. Prolonged QT, Arterial thrombosis, cardiac dysfunction and hemorrhagic events were reported.
Sorafinib	2005	VEGFR	Hepatocellular carcinomas, renal cell carcinomas, thyroid cancers (differentiated)	Diarrhea, fatigue, infection, alopecia, hand-foot skin reaction, rash, weight loss, decreased appetite, nausea, gastrointestinal and abdominal pains, hypertension, and hemorrhage.
Sunitinib	2006	VEGFR	Gastrointestinal stromal tumors, pancreatic neuroendocrine tumors, renal cell carcinomas	Hepatotoxicity, fatigue, asthenia, fever, diarrhea, nausea, mucositis/ stomatitis, vomiting, dyspepsia, abdominal pain, constipation, hypertension, peripheral edema, rash, hand-foot syndrome, skin discoloration, dry skin, hair color changes, altered taste, headache, back pain, arthralgia, extremity pain, cough, dyspnea, anorexia, and bleeding
JAK inhibitors				
Tofacitinib	2012	JAK1/ JAK3	RA, psoriatic arthritis, ulcerative colitis	Series infections, malignancy, upper respiratory tract infections, headache, diarrhea and nasopharyngitis
Baricitinib	2018	JAK1/ JAK2	RA	Series infections, malignancy and thrombosis, upper respiratory tract infections, nausea, herpes simplex, and herpes zoster
Ruxolitinib	2011	JAK1/ JAK2	Myelofibrosis	Thrombocytopenia, anemia, neutropenia bruising, dizziness and headache
Fedratinib	2019	JAK2	Myelofibrosis	Diarrhea, nausea, anemia, and vomiting

Drug	Year of approval	primary target	Indication	Most common adverse reactions and warnings (as mentions in the US prescribing information)
mTOR inhibitors				
Sirolimus	1999	mTOR	Kidney transplant, lymphangioleiomyomatosis	Kidney transplant: peripheral edema, hypertriglyceridemia, hypertension, hypercholesterolemia, creatinine increased, abdominal pain, diarrhea, headache, fever, urinary tract infection, anemia, nausea, arthralgia, pain, and thrombocytopenia Lymphangioleiomyomatosis: stomatitis, diarrhea, abdominal pain, nausea, nasopharyngitis, acne, chest pain, peripheral edema, upper respiratory tract infection, headache, dizziness, myalgia, and hypercholesterolemia
Temsirolimus	2007	mTOR	Advanced renal cell carcinomas	Rash, asthenia, mucositis, nausea, edema, and anorexia, anemia, hyperglycemia, hyperlipemia, hypertriglyceridemia, elevated alkaline phosphatase, elevated serum creatinine, lymphopenia, hypophosphatemia, thrombocytopenia, elevated AST, and leukopenia.
Everolimus	2009	mTOR	HER2-negative breast cancers, pancreatic neuroendocrine tumors, renal cell carcinomas	Advanced RCC: stomatitis, infections, asthenia, fatigue, cough, and diarrhea. SEGA: stomatitis, upper respiratory tract infection, sinusitis, otitis media, and pyrexia.
CDK inhibitors				
Abemaciclib	2017	CDK4/6	breast cancer	Diarrhea, neutropenia, nausea, abdominal pain, infections, fatigue, anemia, leukopenia, decreased appetite, vomiting, headache, alopecia, and thrombocytopenia
Palbociclib	2015	CDK4/6	Estrogen receptor- and HER2-positive breast cancers	Neutropenia, infections, leukopenia, fatigue, nausea, stomatitis, anemia, alopecia, diarrhea, thrombocytopenia, rash, vomiting, decreased appetite, asthenia, and pyrexia
Ribociclib	2017	CDK4/6	Combination therapy for breast cancers	Neutropenia, nausea, fatigue, diarrhea, leukopenia, alopecia, vomiting, constipation, headache and back pain

Table 1.
List of currently approved KIs, their primary targets, identified off-targets, indication and most common adverse reactions in humans as defined in the drug labels.

individual patients [33, 34]. As most of TKIs are metabolized by hepatic cytochrome P450 enzyme system, clinicians should be aware of potential hepatotoxicity with TKIs in patients with liver dysfunction. However, the mechanism for liver toxicity with KIs is not fully clear. Paech et al. [35] studied several approved oncologic KIs (erlotinib, imatinib, lapatinib, and sunitinib) associated with liver toxicity in human hepatocyte cell lines and in isolated mouse liver mitochondria focusing on ATP metabolism. The authors proposed that imatinib (Bcr-Abl TKI) and sunitinib (multiple receptor TKI) induce mitochondrial dysfunction and by inhibiting complex I and/or III of the electron transport chain of the mitochondria required for its function and glycolysis. Lapatinib (HER2 and EGFR TKI) affected mitochondria only weakly but inhibited glycolysis, and erlotinib (EGFR TKI) showed a slight cytotoxicity in both cell models investigated, although it did not affect the mitochondria ATP content in all cell types and did not impair oxidative metabolism. Similar mechanism of inhibition of mitochondrial complex I leading to impaired mitochondrial and myocyte proliferation was published for imatinib and dasatinib (Bcr-Abl and Src TKI) by Bouitbir et al. using C2C12 murine myoblasts and myotubes as well as human rhabdomyosarcoma (RD) cells [36].

In contrast to liver toxicity, it appeared in recent years that TKIs may also prevent or reverse hepatic disease. Accumulating evidence suggests that hepatic stellate cells (HSC) play a pivotal role in hepatic fibrogenesis [37], and that phosphorylation of transcription factors by kinases such as RSK [38] or focal adhesion kinase (FAK) [39] promotes stellate cell activation and survival. Therefore, inhibition of these kinases either as on-targets or off-targets may reduce hepatic disease.

2.3 Hematotoxicity

Hematotoxicity of KIs includes adverse effects on blood-forming organs such as bone marrow or on the constituents of blood, including platelets, leukocytes (white blood cells) and erythrocytes (red blood cells). One particular hematotoxicity caused by KIs is myelosuppression, also known as bone marrow suppression. Myelosuppression is a decrease in bone marrow activity that results in reduced production of blood cells manifested as anemia (decrease in erythrocytes), neutropenia (decrease in leukocytes), or thrombocytopenia (decrease in platelets). VEGF and its receptors are essential for production of mature blood cells [40, 41], as well as are principal regulators of blood vessel formation (angiogenesis) [42]. Accordingly, hematologic toxicities have been observed in clinical studies with several multikinase inhibitors such as VEGFRs KIs (i.e. pazopanib, sorafenib, and sunitinib) [43], although the frequency and severity varies among the different multi-kinase inhibitors, depending on their selectivity and affinity to other kinases [44].

Inhibitors of another two kinases which play roles in hematopoietic activities, FLT3 and mTOR, are also associated with hematotoxicities. A broad range of hematopoietic activities are mediated through interactions of c-Kit ligand (KL) and FLT3 ligand with their receptors: stem cell factor (SCF) and receptor-type tyrosine-protein kinase FLT3, respectively [45]. The signaling through SCF and FLT3 is essential for optimal production of mature haematopoietic cells from stem cells [44]. FLT3 is more critical for the generation of lymphoid progenitors, whereas SCF regulates erythroid and myeloid platelet-derived growth factor (PDGF) progenitor cells. mTOR inhibitors, such as temsirolimus and everolimus, are also associated with a significant increased risk of developing anemia and thrombocytopenia [46], although they have great therapeutic potential in hematologic diseases such as leukemia, lymphoma, myeloma [47]. One possible explanation is that the effect of mTOR inhibition on erythropoiesis could be the antigrowth effect of these KIs on erythrocytes consequently leading to a lower production and decreased size when compared to normal growth [48]. Thus, low selectivity of various KIs towards the above kinases might explain the accompanying hematotoxicity (i.e. imatinib inhibits FLT3 as an off-target).

3. Management of kinase inhibitors associated toxicities

The overall risk for development of the discussed toxicities is different between inhibitors, indications, patients, and patient medical history, and usually the benefit to the patient exceeds the risk associated with development of these adverse events. That is, cardiotoxicity can be managed by routine monitoring via methods such as electroencephalogram, cardiac biomarkers, and blood pressure during the course of treatment, in addition to a comprehensive collection of past medical history and risk factors to identify those at increased risk. When there is a risk for hepatotoxicity, monitoring and management of serum liver chemistry such as elevations of Alanine transaminase (ALT), total bilirubin (TBL) and Alkaline phosphatase (ALP) may identify liver injury during treatment and may suggest reduction in dosage or replacement of KI. Likewise, anemia may be monitored by hematology testing and treatment of iron supplements or erythropoiesis stimulating agents. Regardless, avoiding these side effects via the development of more selective KIs is more advantageous for improving the quality of life of the patients and economy rather than management of the side effects post-marketing. The complex nature of kinase signaling and the challenges of developing selective KIs, suggest that early prediction of selectivity for new molecules and their potential for adverse events in the clinic at preclinical stages may assist and improve the development of future, safer KIs. Proper use of the tool box of preclinical assays as described below may accelerate this goal by identifying and comparing the selectivity of new KIs.

4. Development of selective Protein Kinase Inhibitors

4.1 Methodologies and assays to profile protein kinase inhibitors

Due to the evolving knowledge of the importance of kinases in cell biology and function and their problems of selectivity, multiple methodologies have been developed to profile KIs. Both radiometric and non-radiometric approaches are utilized today. Non-radiometric assays can assess ligand-kinase binding or kinase enzymatic activity. However, the radiometric approach assessing kinase enzymatic activity is still considered the "gold standard". Given the increasing demand for kinase profiling assays and evolution of technology, several companies have developed fee-for-service assays and assay kits [49]. The different methodologies and assays are discussed in the sections below and listed in **Table 2**.

Identifying, quantifying and optimizing the selectivity of compounds became critical for both drug development and development of tool compounds for basic research [19]. Building our knowledge on the selectivity of compounds and creating databases aid in the development of structure-selectivity relationships that will improve rationale design of selective KIs, progress drug discovery and promote inhibitor optimization [65].

Selectivity of KIs is well acknowledged as a challenge in the development of safe drugs and tool compounds. 'Uni-specificity' refers to compounds that inhibit a single kinase more potently than any other kinases. Very few protein KIs demonstrate 'uni-specificity', emphasizing the unresolved issue of selectivity amongst

Assay Type			Fee for service Assay	Reference
Enzymatic Activity Assays	Radioactive methods	Filtration binding assays	Reaction Biology Corporation HotSpot™	[50]
			Promega SignaTECT ™	[51]
		Scintillation proximity assay	Reaction Biology Corporation ^{33}PanQinase™	[50]
	Fluorescent-based assays	Fluorescent intensity assays	DiscoverX ADP Quest™	[52]
			DiscoverX ADP Hunter™	[52]
			BellBrook Labs Transcreener® ADP^2 FI Assay	[53]
		Fluorescent polarization assays	Molecular Device IMAP	[54]
			Bellbrook Labs Transcreener® ADP FP Assay	[53]
		Fluoresccent resonance energy transfer (FRET)	Invitrogen Z'-LYTE	[54]
			PerkinElmer Alpha Kinase assays	[55]
		Time resolved Fluorescence (TRF)	PerkinElmer DELIFA	[56]
		Time resolved Fluorescence resonance Energy transfer (TR-FRET)	Invitrogen LanthaScreen Activity assay	[57]
			Invitrogen Adapta Assay	[58]
			PerkinElmer Lance Ultra kinase Assay	[59]
			Bellbrook Labs Transcreener® ADP TR-FRET Assay	[53]
			Molecular Device IMAP	[54]
		Luciferase reporter Assays	Promega kinase-Glo	[60]
		Electrophoretic Mobility Shift assays	PerkinElmer (formerly Caliper Life Sciences) Nanosyn Assay	[61]
Ligand-kinase binding assays	Competitive binding assay	Immobilized ligand	DiscoverX (formerly Amit Biosciences) KINOMEscan® Assay	[62]
		TR-FRET	Invitrogen's LanthaScreen Eu Kinase binding assay	[63]
	Differential Scanning Fluorimetry			[64]

Table 2.
Kinase inhibitor profiling assays.

protein KIs [20]. Investigating and comparing the selectivity of KIs early in their development is pivotal to developing more selective and consequently safer KIs. Multiple approaches were used to investigate the selectivity of KIs. One approach was to concentrate on the ability of a single KI to inhibit kinases within a specific subfamily due to the similarity in the ATP binding domain. However, importantly, inhibitor type does not guarantee selectivity. Additionally, Anastassiadis et al. [20] demonstrated that a substantial percentage of kinase off-target activity occurred outside the subfamily of interest. For example, 24% of off-target effects of TKIs occurred in the serine/threonine kinase subfamily [20]. Another approach was to focus on the ability of a single KI to inhibit kinases within particular pathways due to shared functionality. A third and most comprehensive approach is to profile KIs against a variety of kinases across the kinome both within and between subfamilies. As technology and assay methodology developed, use of broad screening panels became more common and revealed that compounds historically believed to be selective were in fact not. Today, the best-practice and recommended approach is to screen KIs in different kinase assay formats against multiple related and unrelated kinases. The broad screening panels should be quantitative and systematic with objective criteria to compare between studies. It is important that the assays used are optimized, robust, reliable and standardized for multiple, varied kinases. It is also preferable for practical use of the assays that they are suitable for high-throughput designs and economical [19, 20].

4.2 Enzymatic Activity Assays

4.2.1 Radiometric methods

4.2.1.1 Filtration binding assay

The use of [^{32}P]-or [^{33}P]-ATP in a kinase reaction allows phosphorylation of a substrate peptide or protein to be measured directly. The filtration binding assay approach is the most preferable and the benchmark against which other methodologies are compared. Following a kinase reaction utilizing the radiolabeled ATP molecules, the labelled substrates are bound to capture membranes such as P81 ion exchange filter paper and unchanged ATP/unbound phosphate is washed away. One such assay termed HotSpot™ was developed by Reaction Biology Corporation and Anastassiadis et al. [20] utilized Reaction Biology Corporation's HotSpot™ assay to demonstrate the selectivity of 178 KIs against 300 recombinant protein kinases. Promega's SignaTECT assay operates on a similar principle, however, the SignaTECT assay utilizes biotinylated substrates and a biotin capture membrane to capture the biotinylated substrates with the radiolabeled phosphate for detection [51].

4.2.1.2 Scintillation proximity assay

In order to overcome the necessity for separation and washing steps of the filtration binding assay, the "mix and read" scintillation proximity assays were developed [49]. Reaction Biology Corporation's ^{33}PanQinase™ is an example of a scintillation proximity assay whereby the reaction with [^{33}P]-ATP is performed using microtiter plates coated with scintillant for detection [50]. A variety of radio isotypes can be utilized in a scintillation proximity assay [49].

Despite the advantages of radiometric methodologies such as universality across kinases and low error signal (low false-positive and false-negative rates), the major disadvantage of the radiometric methodology is the specialized waste disposal and safety precautions required for working with radioactive material. As a consequence, non-radioactive methodologies were developed.

4.2.2 Fluorescent based methods

4.2.2.1 Fluorescence Intensity assay

A number of fluorescence intensity assays are available whereby the readout is simply fluorescent intensity (FI). DiscoverX ADP Hunter™ and ADP Quest™FI assays use linked reactions that use ADP, pyruvate kinase, pyruvate oxidase and horseradish peroxidase to convert a fluorescent dye precursor (ADHP (10-Acetyl-3,7-dihydroxyphenoxazine) to fluorescent resorufin, the source of the fluorescent intensity signal [52]. Bellbrook Labs Transcreener® ADP FI Assay measures ADP levels. This is accomplished by utilizing an IRDye® QC-1 quencher conjugated to an anti-ADP antibody to quench the signal from an ADP Alexa Fluor® 594 tracer. Once ADP is produced, ADP displaces the fluorescent tracer allowing detection of the fluorescent signal from the fluorescent tracer [53].

4.2.2.2 Fluorescent polarization assays

Exciting molecules with polarized light promotes rotational movement. The speed of the rotational movement depends on the molecular weight of the compound. That is, high molecular weight molecules rotate slower than low molecular weight molecules. Molecular Device developed a "mix and read" FP assay whereby following kinase reaction a fluorescently labelled, phosphorylated substrate binds to a large nanoparticle increasing the molecular weight, decreasing rotational speed and increasing the polarization of the phosphorylated peptide or protein [54]. However, false-positive and false-negatives have been reported utilizing the FP methodology [49].

4.2.2.3 Fluorescent resonance energy transfer (FRET)

Fluorescent resonance energy transfer (FRET) relies on the transfer of energy between donor and acceptor molecules that occurs when the two molecules come into close proximity and following excitation of the donor molecule. Many companies have utilized this technology to develop assays for kinase profiling including Invitrogen's Z'-LYTE Kinase Assay utilized in their SelectScreen Kinase Profiling Service. In invitrogen's Z'-LYTE Kinase Assay, two fluorescent proteins that make up FRET donor and acceptor molecules are added to substrates, then following the kinase reaction, the non-phosphorylated substrates are cleaved by a protease interrupting the energy transfer between the donor and acceptor fluorophores. Therefore, the emission wavelength differs depending on if the substrate was phosphorylated or not. The assay relies on identification of the amino acid sequence of the relevant substrate and has been validated for more than 200 kinases [49, 66].

4.2.2.4 Time-resolved fluorescence (TRF)

Time-resolved fluorescence (TRF) involves the use of fluorophores that decay over a longer period of time than traditionally used fluorophores and the decay following light excitation of these fluorophores can be monitored as a function of time. Lanthanide chelates such as Europium, Samarium and Terbium are examples of such non-traditional fluorophores with long decay times. PerkinElmer's DELFIA® assay is available as a TRF assay that utilizes lanthanide chelate tagged antibodies to detect phosphorylated substrates [49, 56].

4.2.2.5 Time-resolved fluorescence resonance energy transfer (TR-FRET)

A time-resolved fluorescence resonance energy transfer (TR-FRET) assay combines the principle of FRET with donor and acceptor molecules with TRF whereby one of the molecules is a fluorophore with an extended decay time [49]. For example, in addition to Invitrogen's Z'-LYTE FRET assay, Invitrogen also offer several TR-FRET assays (LanthaScreen Activity assay, LanthaScreen Eu Kinase binding assay [discussed below in Section 1.3.2] and Adapta Assay). The Adapta Assay utilizes a Europium-labeled anti-ADP antibody and an Alexa Fluor® 647 labeled ADP tracer to examine ADP levels following a kinase reaction. Without the presence of ADP, the anti-ADP antibody and ADP tracer bind to create the TR-FRET signal. ADP disrupts the binding of the antibody and tracer reducing the signal. Alternatively, the LanthaScreen® activity assay involves a fluorophore-labelled substrate that when phosphorylated is bound by Terbium-labeled antibody to generate the FRET signal [57, 58]. Similarly, PerkinElmer's Lance® Ultra kinase assay utilizes U*Light*™-labeled substrate that when phosphorylated is bound by Europium-labeled antibody to generate the FRET signal. Similar to the Z'-LYTE Kinase Assay, the LanthaScreen Activity assay and Lance® Ultra kinase assay both rely on identification of the amino acid sequence of the relevant substrate [59].

4.2.3 Luciferase reporter assay

Cell-based luciferase reporter assays that produce bioluminescence are common to monitor the activity of cellular processes. Cell-based luciferase reporter assays require luciferin, luciferase enzyme and sometimes ATP. The Firefly luciferase enzyme converts luciferin into oxiluciferin in the presence of ATP emitting a light photon. As the conversion of luciferin to oxiluciferin relies on ATP, the luciferase enzyme can be used to detect the amount of ATP following a kinase reaction and the amount of luminescence positively correlates with the amount of ATP [49, 67]. An example of a commercially available luciferase assay for kinase profiling is Promega's Kinase-Glo® platform [60].

It is also important to differentiate when utilizing a luciferase reporter assay between compounds that legitimately inhibit a kinase from compounds that interfere with the assay itself. That is, luciferase itself may be targeted by KIs [67]. Dranchak et al. [67] investigated the ability 367 compounds in the GSK published protein kinase inhibitor set to inhibit two commonly used types of luciferase enzymes (firefly luciferase [FLuc; ATP-dependent] and renilla renififormis luciferase [RLuc; ATP-independent]). Approximately 6% of the KIs inhibited FLuc activity whereas approximately 0.5% inhibited RLuc activity. Therefore, the specific luciferase utilized and the potential interactions of KIs with the luciferase should be taken into consideration when choosing an appropriate assay platform for kinase profiling using luciferase [67].

4.2.4 Electrophoretic Mobility Shift Assays

Phosphorylation of a substrate causes an increase in the negative charge of the substrate. As a consequence, phosphorylated substrates can be separated and detected using electrophoretic technologies. The Caliper Life Sciences' Nanosyn

Assay takes advantage of these properties of phosphorylated substrates (usually fluorescently labelled peptides and proteins) and utilizes a microfluidic chip for the assay reaction and electrophoretic detection [49, 61, 68]. Elkins et al. [68] utilized this assay to examine the selectivity of the GSK published protein kinase inhibitor set against 224 recombinant kinases with a 50% inhibition threshold and identified that there are different kinases targeted by multiple compounds, kinases not inhibited by any of the compounds and kinases inhibited by only one compound.

4.3 Ligand-kinase binding assays

Measuring the effect of ligands on the enzymatic activity of kinases has traditionally been the "go to" approach. However, enzymatic activity assays require individual optimization in order to receive an acceptable signal-to-noise ratio as well as identification of upstream signaling partners and applicable substrates. The requirements for optimization of enzymatic activity assays cannot always be met and individual optimization of the assays for each kinase can be costly and time consuming. Therefore, binding assays were developed utilizing different technologies including competitive binding assays and differential scanning fluorimetry to facilitate high-throughput kinase profiling [64, 69]. Although suitable to enable high-throughput screening, ligand-kinase binding assays do not always predict enzymatic activity of a compound with the particular kinase [20, 69].

4.3.1 Competitive binding assays

One option for a competitive binding assay is Invitrogen's LanthaScreen Eu Kinase binding assay using TR-FRET technology as described in Section 4.2.2.5. That is, the assay operates whereby a Europium-labeled antibody is targeted against a tagged kinase and an Alexa Fluor® 647 labeled substrate are used to generate the FRET signal. Inhibitor binding to the kinase prevents substrate binding and disrupts the FRET signal [63].

An alternative approach is the DiscoverX's KINOMEscan assay utilizing immobilized ligands [62]. The KINOMEscan platform was originally published by Ambit Biosciences. The KINOMEscan platform involves phage or DNA tagged kinases and immobilized ligands. The ligands are biotinylated and then bound to streptavidin-coated magnetic beads attached to solid supports. The immobilized ligands compete with compounds for binding to the kinase. ATP-binding and allosteric KIs can compete with the immobilized ligands. Kinase that is unbound to the immobilized ligand is removed via wash steps. The amount of kinase bound to the immobilized ligands is then quantified using qPCR identifying the phage or DNA tag attached to the kinase. The assay has been validated for more than 450 kinases (wild-type and mutant) [69–71]. Utilizing this technique, Davis et al. [69] screened 72 KIs and demonstrated that type II inhibitors are more selective than type I inhibitors with the majority of type II inhibitors demonstrating binding to 20% or less of the total kinases screened. However, a KI belonging to the type II class does not guarantee selectivity with a subset of type II inhibitors binding to 40–50% of kinases screened [69].

4.3.2 Differential Scanning Fluorimetry

Upon binding of a ligand to a protein, such as a kinase, the thermal properties of the protein stabilize and the melting temperature increases. The unfolded, unbound kinase that is not stabilized is detected by a dye that binds to unfolded proteins and fluoresces. This methodology is termed differential scanning fluorimetry (DSF).

SYPRO orange is a suitable fluorescent dye for this application due to the high signal-to-noise ratio and comparably high excitation wavelength [64, 72]. Fedorov, Niesen and Knapp [64] demonstrated that the data generated using the KINOMEscan assay developed by Ambit Biosciences and described above (Section 4.3.1) highly correlated with their data generated using DSF with an r^2 value of 0.949. A major advantage of the thermal stability shift methodology is that knowledge of the amino acid sequence of the substrate or kinase is not required and specialized antibodies are also not required [64]. Additionally, Anastassiadis, et al. [20] compared the DSF method to Reaction Biology Corporation's radiometric method and found a significant correlation between the two methodologies. However, the DSF method did demonstrate false-positives and false-negatives and thus emphasizing that binding does not necessarily predict enzymatic activity [20].

4.4 Computational analysis

Computational kinase selectivity profiling methods can be used to predict the selectivity of KIs and rationally design KIs with desired profiles across a large number of kinases and avoid the limitations of activity and binding assays. However, computational approaches are dependent on the quality of the available structure–activity data or require extensive computational analysis [73]. Improved computational approaches take advantage of the conservational nature of the kinome and shared binding patterns of KIs as well as profiling data generated for multiple kinases across the classes and kinome and kinase 3D structures. Kinase inhibition profiling data including both positive and negative (little or no effect) data are invaluable to the evaluation of computational approaches for predicting KI selectivity [74]. The large volume of data generated to date paved the way for the development of machine learning and artificial intelligence approaches that allow for prediction of results for KIs and kinases not included in the dataset [19, 73–75]. With the accumulation of structure–activity data over the years, the literature has been minded to create both commercially and publically available databases with data from diverse sources such as ChEMBL, Kinase SARfari and GVK Biosciences kinase inhibitor database. The kinase-inhibitor profiling panels already discussed here such as those generated by Karaman [70], Anastassiadis [20] and Davis [69] as well as other databases such as the 3D structures available in PDB were also used to generate numerous computational approaches. The size of the gatekeeper residue, hydrogen and covalent bonds, the flexibility of the hinge loop connecting kinase domains as well as kinase-inhibitor data were all used to generate computational approaches. The KI data can be represented either as binary yes-no or weighted by affinity or inhibitory activity and can be used to generate connectivity maps to predict either kinases, KIs or diseases [74]. Lo et al. [73] developed a computational approach based on searching for structural similarity of the ligand binding sites and determining a PocketFEATURE score (PFS). Specifically, a kinase database entitled 'KinomeFEATURE' of approximately 2850 kinase structures was constructed to predict selectivity of 15 known KIs with greater than 90% accuracy. Therefore, computational approaches are becoming more widely used and useful for the purpose of predicting selectivity and rationally design KIs [73].

4.5 Quantification of selectivity

In order to aid in the ability to compare data between studies and assay methodologies to identify and compare the selectivity of inhibitors, different quantitative measures of selectivity have been developed. These measures involve condensing large datasets into single values for each inhibitor. Such measures include the selectivity score, Gini coefficient score and selectivity entropy score described below. However, the selectivity score for a particular KI takes into consideration all kinases in a dataset and rely upon the size and diversity of the kinases in the dataset [76].

4.5.1 Selectivity score

In order to generate a selectivity score for a particular inhibitor, the number of kinases bound by this specific inhibitor with $K_d$or IC_{50} values that meet pre-defined threshold criteria should be divided by the total number of distinct kinases screened in a specific assay [20, 69, 70]. The predefined threshold can be a specific concentration e.g. 3 μM [S(3 μM)] or percentage e.g. 50% [S(50%)]. For example, Karaman et al. [70] from Amit Biosciences utilized the KINOMEscan to screen 38 KIs against 317 kinases and calculated selectivity scores S(3 μM) and S(100 nM) whereby K_d < 3 μM and K_d < 100 nM, respectively. Via the use of the selectivity score, Karaman et al. [70] showed that the compounds screened demonstrated a fairly even distribution of selectivity scores from 0.01 to 0.57 (1–57%).However, Karaman et al. [70] also demonstrated that the composition of the kinases in the screened database significantly affected the outcome. That is, the selectivity score varied greatly by adjusting the number of kinases screened and randomly selecting kinases preserved the results better than a systematic selection. Karaman et al. [70] also described a selectivity score to describe off-target affinities whereby a ratio of the K_d for the off-target to the K_d of the primary target is generated and then the number of ratios below 10 is then divided by the total number of distinct kinases assayed. This selectivity score was also termed S(10x). Later, Davis et al. [69] (Amit Biosciences) also used the KINOMEscan to screen 72 KIs against 442 kinases and demonstrated that the majority (64%; 46 out of 72) of inhibitors bound to <20% of the total distinct kinases screened by them (totaling 386) with a S(3 μM) score of <0.2.

The selectivity score is not limited to the assay type or assay technology facilitating comparisons between compounds, studies and assays [70]. The selectivity score is, however, dependent on the threshold set for defining the score such as 3 μM vs. 100 nM or 50% vs. 70% inhibition [20].

4.5.2 Gini Coefficient

The Gini coefficient has been described as a less arbitrary tool for evaluating selectivity compared to the selectivity score described above as the Gini coefficient does not rely on defining a threshold value. To calculate the Gini coefficient, the % inhibition of a compound at a single concentration is rank ordered, summed and normalized to generate a plot of rank order vs. fraction of cumulative effect of each target. Then, the deviation from the linear plot is calculated and a greater deviation from the linear plot indicates a less specific compound. A Gini score of 1 indicates an inhibitor that targets one kinase whereas a score of 0 indicates a compound that equally inhibits all kinases screened. Even though the Gini coefficient does not rely on a defined threshold, the coefficient relies on the single concentration tested and is thus inherently limited [20, 76].

4.5.3 Selectivity Entropy Value

Following the use of selectivity scores and the Gini coefficient to quantitatively describe inhibitor selectivity, Uitdehaag and Zaman [76] introduced the entropy value to overcome the limitations of the selectivity score and Gini coefficient score.

The entropy value was previously utilized in a diverse range of fields such as thermodynamics and chemistry, and it is based on the concept that inhibitor binding to multiple kinases will assume a Boltzmann distribution [76]. The entropy equation utilized by Uitdehaag and Zaman [76] involves 5 steps based on the association constant (K_a, the inverse of the K_d or IC_{50} values).

A resulting selectivity entropy (S_{sel}) value of 0 indicates an inhibitor that targets one kinase and the higher the S_{sel} the less specific the compound is for the kinases profiled. Uitdehaag and Zaman [76] compared the selectivity entropy value to the selectivity score S(3 μM), K_a-Gini (Gini scores based on association constants), S(10x) and partition index (not outlined in this review) for data generated using the KINOMEscan compared to a radioactive filter binding enzymatic activity assay by Millipore. The two methodologies produced highly correlated data using the selectivity entropy score, S(3 μM) and K_a-Gini with r^2 correlation values of 0.93, 0.92 and 0.99, respectively, showing that these three scores are relatively robust. Uitdehaag and Zaman [76] also demonstrated that type II and III inhibitors are more selective than type I inhibitors consistent with the conclusions drawn by Davis et al. [69] using the selectivity score S(3 μM).

4.6 Graphical representation of selectivity

For qualitative rather than quantitative analysis of a compound selectivity, different graphical representations have been used to demonstrate the interaction of a compound with the whole kinome or kinase panel in the assay. Interaction maps and heat maps have been used to represent and compare compound selectivity. Interaction maps are based on the phylogenetic tree. In interaction maps, a circle is overlaid on a kinase in the kinase phylogenetic tree representing interaction of the compound with the kinase and the size of the circle represents potency. That is, the larger the circle the higher affinity the compound has for the kinase [68, 70, 76]. Graphical representations allow for visual rankings of selectivity and these visual observations should align with any quantitative measure chosen [76].

4.7 Cell-based vs. Cell-free selectivity assays

Regardless if binding or enzymatic activity assays are chosen, it is important to understand that cell-free in vitro assays may not reflect the activity in cellular systems. As such, it is recommended to follow-up cell-free in vitro selectivity assays with cell-based selectivity assays in vitro or in vivo animal model systems [65, 70, 77].

Cell-based assays are more complex than cell-free based assays and this complexity contributes to the discrepancies between the assays. One source of complexity in cell-based assays is the fact that the phosphorylation state in cells relies on the balance between phosphorylation of proteins by kinases and de-phosphorylation of proteins by phosphatases and this can lower the required concentration of KIs for kinase inhibition. Additionally, our understanding of phosphatase systems and their regulators is more limited. Moreover, sensitivities differ when assessing different cellular activities such as calcium release, IL-2 secretion or proliferation of T-cells [65] as measures for enzymatic reaction and selectivity.

An important difference between cell-based and cell-free selectivity assays is that in the cell-based assay the KI must penetrate the cell membrane and the cellular compartments in order for the inhibitor to reach its target. Different factors determine if a KI reaches its target within a cell. A KI can penetrate a cell either via a diffusion concentration gradient or active transport and a KI can also be actively pumped out of cells via efflux mechanisms. Size, lipophilic properties, aqueous solubility, plasma membrane partitioning and plasma protein binding, for in vivo assays, will impact the ability of a KI to reach its target within a cell. It is important to test the KI once the compound reaches steady state within the cell and therefore it is routine practice to pre-incubate cells with the KI prior to performing a cell-based kinase activity assay [65].

The metabolic activity and ATP concentration in cells will also affect inhibitor activity within cells. In order to compare IC_{50} values to K_d values, it is best practice to use ATP concentrations equal to the Michaelis constant for ATP ($K_{M, ATP}$) for the particular kinase in an enzymatic assay based on the Cheng-Prusoff equation: $IC_{50} = K_i(1 + [ATP]/K_{M, ATP})$, whereby K_i is the dissociation constant. However, ATP concentrations are generally higher in cellular systems compared to the $K_{M, ATP}$ and differences in ATP concentrations may be a source of discrepancy between cell-based and cell-free selectivity assays [65, 76].

An additional potential difference between cell-based and cell-free selectivity assays is that some cell-free screening panels use truncated forms of the kinases and interactions between a kinase and inhibitor may differ in the setting of the full-length kinase.

The conformational state of the kinase should also be taken into consideration when assaying the interaction with a KI as many kinases can adopt different conformational states. For example, inhibitors that bind to the inactive state of a kinase can stabilize the kinase in this state which may not occur in a cell-free assay with a truncated form of the kinase [20].

5. Overcoming toxicity with more selective kinase inhibitors

The first generation of KIs, including imatinib, which was the first KI approved by the FDA in 2001 for patients with chronic myeloid leukemia (CML), demonstrated acceptable toxicity profiles in oncology patients compared with traditional chemotherapeutic agents, as well as comparable efficacy even though the first generation KIs were not highly selective. However, the acceptable toxicity and risk–benefit ratio are higher for oncology patients than for patients with conditions that are not severely debilitating or life-threatening such as chronic inflammatory disease [78]. Therefore, there is a growing need to overcome lack of selectivity and off-target toxicities with newly developed KIs for different indications.

An example of overcoming toxicity by improving selectivity and by lowering affinity for off-targets is coming from the JAK family of non-receptor tyrosine kinases that has gained great interest as therapeutic targets. The JAKs transduce signals from a multitude of cytokines and growth factors via the JAK–STAT (Signal Transducers and Activators of Transcription) pathway and are involved in various inflammatory and autoimmune diseases [79, 80]. Currently, there are four JAK inhibitors approved for clinical use: tofacitinib (for RA, psoriatic arthritis, ulcerative colitis), baricitinib (for RA), ruxolitinib and fedratinib (for myelofibrosis). These JAK inhibitors demonstrate that improved selectivity results in more favorable safety profile, and also emphasize that the existence of off-target binding does not automatically predict unfavorable safety profiles because the off-target activity plays a major role. That is, lower activity of these JAK inhibitors on their off-targets result in lower toxicity. Since JAK inhibitors block downstream signaling of a variety of cytokines relevant for normal physiology, various severe adverse effects were often predicted for these inhibitors. However, clinical trials of tofacitinib have shown an acceptable safety profile, with infection and cytopenias (due to the blockage of myelopoietic growth factor signaling through JAK2) being the major adverse events, and without any increased risk of developing malignancies [81].

Likewise, the selective JAK1/JAK2 inhibitor baricitinib, which offers an effective treatment for RA, demonstrates little effect on hematology parameters, with uncommon neutropenia (<1% patients) and no higher risk of infection [82]. A reduction in natural killer (NK) cell numbers was observed in some patients, but there was no evident association between the low NK cell count and the incidence of infections. Ruxolitinib is another potent JAK1/JAK2 inhibitor demonstrating dose-dependent inhibition of the JAK2/STAT signaling and inhibition of cell growth that is dependent on JAK2 activation, with a sixfold selectivity for JAK1/JAK2 over Tyk2 and approximately a 130-fold selectivity for JAK1/JAK2 over JAK3 [83]. Despite this high selectivity, thrombocytopenia and anemia are side effects of ruxolitinib which can be dose- or even treatment-limiting adverse events and patients who discontinue ruxolitinib have miserable outcomes, making this situation an area of significant unmet need [84, 85]. Recently, fedratinib was approved by the FDA as a different drug for myelofibrosis overcoming some of the toxicities and resistance observed in ruxolitinib-refractory patients [86]. Fedratinib is selective for JAK2 over other JAKs and the common side effects reported with this drug include anemia, gastrointestinal symptoms, and elevations in liver transaminases [87]. Fedratinib also has a black box warning for encephalopathy, although this occurred only in about 1% of the treated patients [87]. Overall, increasing selectivity of JAK inhibitors may decrease the side effect burden on the patient but this cannot be avoided completely due their mechanism of action on important signal transduction pathways.

In an attempt to develop more selective second-generation JAK inhibitors, there are more than 20 other JAK inhibitors undergoing clinical trials, with varying selectivity profiles, for a variety of autoimmune diseases, including psoriasis, alopecia areata, ankylosing spondylitis and lupus [87]. Within the JAK family, JAK3 inhibitors are emerging as potential targets for the design of more selective KIs. JAK3 is a potential target for inflammatory diseases and has a more defined function than other JAKs, which participate in multiple cellular processes. JAK3 associates only with the common γ-chain receptor, and it is expressed selectively in lymphoid and myeloid cells. Consequently, selective JAK3 inhibition may be beneficial in suppressing inflammatory responses with less off-target effects and markedly reduced adverse effects [80]. The main concern that has arisen recently with JAK inhibitors from pharmacovigilance (real-world data analysis) is a higher risk of thromboembolism [88, 89]. Conflicting data indicates that higher thromboembolic risk may be related to the specificity of JAK inhibitor action, such that preferentially blocking one signaling pathway upsets the balance between pro and anti-thrombotic activities [90]. It could be that thromboembolic complications are not a general class effect of JAK inhibitors, but might be related to inhibition of a specific JAK, aging and mutations in JAKs and the patient clinical history.

Even though the threshold for acceptable toxicities is higher for oncology patients due to the higher risk–benefit ratio that is tolerated, effort continues to be invested into producing more selective anti-cancer KI treatments with fewer side effects because these drugs fail in clinical trials due to overt toxicity. Promising and selective anti-cancer agents are cyclin-dependent kinases (CDKs) inhibitors. CDKs are important players in the regulation of cell division and proliferation, and numerous drugs that target CDKs have been developed to treat cancers over the past 20 years. The clinical trials with the first CDK inhibitors were discontinued due to severe toxicities. These toxicities were related to the low selectivity of the CDK inhibitors, since CDKs such as CK1 and CDK2 that are essential for maintaining the growth and function of normal cells were also inhibited [91]. More recently approved CDK inhibitors for the treatment of patients with breast cancer, including palbociclib, ribociclib, and abemaciclib, which exhibit selectivity for CDK4/6 over other CDKs, are associated with a lower numbers of life-threatening side effects [92]. These inhibitors do not have cross reactivity with other CDKs nor with other kinases in general and therefore have an improved safety profile [93]. Other selective CDK inhibitors are currently under development [94].

6. Conclusion and future perspectives

Hundreds of diseases including various cancers, Alzheimer's disease and auto-immune are associated with kinase mediated phosphorylation of proteins, and therefore discovery of selective KIs is still an urgent need. Selectivity is a known challenge for the development of KIs as safe therapeutics and as reliable tool compounds to investigate biological activities. Therefore, it is important to investigate the selectivity of KIs against kinase panels as well as against other targets such as other enzymes, ion channels and receptors. As a consequence, the technologies for assessing the selectivity of KIs are constantly evolving and have become increasingly sophisticated. In particular, the development of techniques that measure inhibitor profiles in environments that mimic human physiology would provide more reliable and human relevant results on the KI selectivity. Optimization of KIs, either by structure based drug-design, identifying and targeting allosteric sites or enhancing affinity for the on-target kinase, improves selectivity, and in general more selective KIs were shown to have more favorable safety profiles. The recently approved CDK and JAK inhibitors provide a proof of concept that safer and more effective KIs can be developed for both oncology indications and non-oncology indications such as chronic inflammatory diseases. Recent progress in nanomedicine and targeted therapy offers improvement of drug efficacy, and allow for specific delivery of TKIs to the diseased cells using special nanocarriers, thereby reducing the incidence of adverse events [95]. Yet, TKI-nanomedicines are in the initial stages of development and, although they have great potential, they still have a long way ahead of them. Overall, achieving improved target selectivity and reduced off-target-mediated toxicity using efficient compound screening and profiling technologies, providing targeted therapies and overcoming resistance will further pave the way for novel, selective and safe KIs as promising therapeutics in oncology and beyond.

Acknowledgements

We would like to thank Dr. Efrat Rubinstein for critically reviewing this manuscript, and Dr. Dvir Doron for assisting with visualization of the crystal structures of selected kinases.

DOI: http://dx.doi.org/10.5772/intechopen.98640

Author details

Moran Grossman* and Elaine Adler
Global Research and Development, Teva Pharmaceutical Industries Ltd., Netanya, Israel

*Address all correspondence to: moran.grossman@teva.co.il

References

[1] Ardito, F., et al., *The crucial role of protein phosphorylation in cell signaling and its use as targeted therapy (Review).* Int J Mol Med, 2017. **40**(2): p. 271-280.

[2] Duong-Ly, K. C. and J. R. Peterson, *The human kinome and kinase inhibition as a therapeutic strategy.* Curr Protoc Pharmacol, 2013. **Chapter 2**: p. Unit2 9.

[3] Tsai, C. J. and R. Nussinov, *The molecular basis of targeting protein kinases in cancer therapeutics.* Semin Cancer Biol, 2013. **23**(4): p. 235-242.

[4] Zarrin, A. A., et al., *Kinase inhibition in autoimmunity and inflammation.* Nat Rev Drug Discov, 2021. **20**(1): p. 39-63.

[5] Gaestel, M., A. Kotlyarov, and M. Kracht, *Targeting innate immunity protein kinase signalling in inflammation.* Nat Rev Drug Discov, 2009. **8**(6): p. 480-499.

[6] Wagey, R. T. and C. Krieger, *Abnormalities of protein kinases in neurodegenerative diseases.* Prog Drug Res, 1998. **51**: p. 133-183.

[7] Roskoski, R., Jr., *Properties of FDA-approved small molecule protein kinase inhibitors: A 2020 update.* Pharmacol Res, 2020. **152**: p. 104609.

[8] Benn, C. L. and L. A. Dawson, *Clinically Precedented Protein Kinases: Rationale for Their Use in Neurodegenerative Disease.* Front Aging Neurosci, 2020. **12**: p. 242.

[9] Bhullar, K. S., et al., *Kinase-targeted cancer therapies: progress, challenges and future directions.* Mol Cancer, 2018. **17**(1): p. 48.

[10] Ferguson, F. M. and N. S. Gray, *Kinase inhibitors: the road ahead.* Nat Rev Drug Discov, 2018. **17**(5): p. 353-377.

[11] Dar, A. C. and K. M. Shokat, *The evolution of protein kinase inhibitors from antagonists to agonists of cellular signaling.* Annu Rev Biochem, 2011. **80**: p. 769-795.

[12] Baier A, Szyszka R., *Compounds from Natural Sources as Protein Kinase.* Biomolecules. , 2020. **10**(11): p. 1546.

[13] Schrödinger, Inc. *Maestro*. 2021 [cited 2021 21 March, 2021]; Available from: https://www.schrodinger.com/maestro.

[14] Kufareva, I. and R. Abagyan, *Type-II kinase inhibitor docking, screening, and profiling using modified structures of active kinase states.* J Med Chem, 2008. **51**(24): p. 7921-7932.

[15] Foda, Z. H. and M. A. Seeliger, *Kinase inhibitors: an allosteric add-on.* Nat Chem Biol, 2014. **10**(10): p. 796-797.

[16] Panicker, R. C., et al., *Allosteric Small-Molecule Serine/Threonine Kinase Inhibitors.* Adv Exp Med Biol, 2019. **1163**: p. 253-278.

[17] Wu, P., M. H. Clausen, and T. E. Nielsen, *Allosteric small-molecule kinase inhibitors.* Pharmacol Ther, 2015. **156**: p. 59-68.

[18] Munoz, L., *Non-kinase targets of protein kinase inhibitors.* Nat Rev Drug Discov, 2017. **16**(6): p. 424-440.

[19] Smyth, L. A. and I. Collins, *Measuring and interpreting the selectivity of protein kinase inhibitors.* J Chem Biol, 2009. **2**(3): p. 131-151.

[20] Anastassiadis, T., et al., *Comprehensive assay of kinase catalytic activity reveals features of kinase inhibitor selectivity.* Nat Biotechnol, 2011. **29**(11): p. 1039-1045.

[21] Fauvel, B. and A. Yasri, *Antibodies directed against receptor tyrosine kinases:*

current and future strategies to fight cancer. MAbs, 2014. **6**(4): p. 838-851.

[22] Holcmann, M. and M. Sibilia, *Mechanisms underlying skin disorders induced by EGFR inhibitors.* Mol Cell Oncol, 2015. **2**(4): p. e1004969.

[23] Fakih, M. and M. Vincent, *Adverse events associated with anti-EGFR therapies for the treatment of metastatic colorectal cancer.* Curr Oncol, 2010. **17 Suppl 1**: p. S18-S30.

[24] Brand, T. M., M. Iida, and D. L. Wheeler, *Molecular mechanisms of resistance to the EGFR monoclonal antibody cetuximab.* Cancer Biol Ther, 2011. **11**(9): p. 777-792.

[25] Udupa, K. S., et al., *Differential Toxicities of Tyrosine Kinase Inhibitors in the Management of Metastatic Lung Cancer.* Indian J Med Paediatr Oncol, 2017. **38**(1): p. 15-17.

[26] Shah, R. R. and D. R. Shah, *Safety and Tolerability of Epidermal Growth Factor Receptor (EGFR) Tyrosine Kinase Inhibitors in Oncology.* Drug Saf, 2019. **42**(2): p. 181-198.

[27] Lamore, S. D., et al., *Cardiovascular Toxicity Induced by Kinase Inhibitors: Mechanisms and Preclinical Approaches.* Chem Res Toxicol, 2020. **33**(1): p. 125-136.

[28] Fuller, S. J., et al., *Cardiac protein kinases: the cardiomyocyte kinome and differential kinase expression in human failing hearts.* Cardiovasc Res, 2015. **108**(1): p. 87-98.

[29] Force, T., D. S. Krause, and R. A. Van Etten, *Molecular mechanisms of cardiotoxicity of tyrosine kinase inhibition.* Nat Rev Cancer, 2007. **7**(5): p. 332-344.

[30] Touyz, R. M. and J. Herrmann, *Cardiotoxicity with vascular endothelial growth factor inhibitor therapy.* NPJ Precis Oncol, 2018. **2**: p. 13.

[31] Sciarretta, S., et al., *New Insights Into the Role of mTOR Signaling in the Cardiovascular System.* Circ Res, 2018. **122**(3): p. 489-505.

[32] Shi, Q., et al., *Recent advances in understanding the hepatotoxicity associated with protein kinase inhibitors.* Expert Opin Drug Metab Toxicol, 2020. **16**(3): p. 217-226.

[33] Aqsa, A., et al., *Sunitinib-Induced Acute Liver Failure.* Case Rep Gastroenterol, 2021. **15**(1): p. 17-21.

[34] Ivanyi, P., et al., *Hepatic toxicity during regorafenib treatment in patients with metastatic gastrointestinal stromal tumors.* Mol Clin Oncol, 2020. **13**(6): p. 72.

[35] Paech, F., J. Bouitbir, and S. Krahenbuhl, *Hepatocellular Toxicity Associated with Tyrosine Kinase Inhibitors: Mitochondrial Damage and Inhibition of Glycolysis.* Front Pharmacol, 2017. **8**: p. 367.

[36] Bouitbir, J., et al., *Imatinib and Dasatinib Provoke Mitochondrial Dysfunction Leading to Oxidative Stress in C2C12 Myotubes and Human RD Cells.* Front Pharmacol, 2020. **11**: p. 1106.

[37] Qu, K., et al., *Tyrosine kinase inhibitors: friends or foe in treatment of hepatic fibrosis?* Oncotarget, 2016. **7**(41): p. 67650-67660.

[38] Buck, M., et al., *C/EBPbeta phosphorylation by RSK creates a functional XEXD caspase inhibitory box critical for cell survival.* Mol Cell, 2001. **8**(4): p. 807-816.

[39] Zhao, X. K., et al., *Focal Adhesion Kinase Regulates Hepatic Stellate Cell Activation and Liver Fibrosis.* Sci Rep, 2017. **7**(1): p. 4032.

[40] Shibuya, M., *Vascular endothelial growth factor and its receptor system: physiological functions in angiogenesis and*

pathological roles in various diseases. J Biochem, 2013. **153**(1): p. 13-19.

[41] Gerber, H. P. and N. Ferrara, *The role of VEGF in normal and neoplastic hematopoiesis.* J Mol Med (Berl), 2003. **81**(1): p. 20-31.

[42] Ferrara, N., *The role of VEGF in the regulation of physiological and pathological angiogenesis.* EXS, 2005(94): p. 209-231.

[43] Schutz, F. A., Y. Je, and T. K. Choueiri, *Hematologic toxicities in cancer patients treated with the multi-tyrosine kinase sorafenib: a meta-analysis of clinical trials.* Crit Rev Oncol Hematol, 2011. **80**(2): p. 291-300.

[44] Kumar, R., et al., *Myelosuppression and kinase selectivity of multikinase angiogenesis inhibitors.* Br J Cancer, 2009. **101**(10): p. 1717-1723.

[45] Lyman, S. D. and S. E. Jacobsen, *c-kit ligand and Flt3 ligand: stem/progenitor cell factors with overlapping yet distinct activities.* Blood, 1998. **91**(4): p. 1101-1134.

[46] Xu, J. and D. Tian, *Hematologic toxicities associated with mTOR inhibitors temsirolimus and everolimus in cancer patients: a systematic review and meta-analysis.* Curr Med Res Opin, 2014. **30**(1): p. 67-74.

[47] Feng, Y., et al., *The Role of mTOR Inhibitors in Hematologic Disease: From Bench to Bedside.* Front Oncol, 2020. **10**: p. 611690.

[48] Diekmann, F., et al., *mTOR inhibition and erythropoiesis: microcytosis or anaemia?* Nephrol Dial Transplant, 2012. **27**(2): p. 537-41.

[49] Ma, H., S. Deacon, and K. Horiuchi, *The challenge of selecting protein kinase assays for lead discovery optimization.* Expert Opin Drug Discov, 2008. **3**(6): p. 607-621.

[50] Biology, Reaction. *Kinase Screening*. 2021 March 23, 2021]; Available from: https://www.reactionbiology.com/services/target-specific-assays/kinase-assays/kinase-screening.

[51] Corporation, Promega. *SignaTECT® Protein Kinase Assay Systems*. 2021 March 23, 2021]; Available from: https://www.promega.com/products/cell-signaling/kinase-assays-and-kinase-biology/signatect-protein-kinase-assay-systems/?catNum=V7470.

[52] Products, Eurofins DiscoverX. *ADP Accumulation Assays*. 2020 March 23, 2021]; Available from: https://www.discoverx.com/technologies-platforms/fluorescence-intensity-technology/adp-accumulation-assay-platform.

[53] Labs, BellBrook. *Transcreener® ADP^2 Kinase Assay Kits*. 2019 March 23, 2021]; Available from: https://www.bellbrooklabs.com/products/transcreener-hts-assays/kinase-assays/.

[54] Molecular Devices, LLC. *Enzyme - IMAP Assays*. 2021 March 23, 2021]; Available from: https://www.moleculardevices.com/products/assay-kits/enzyme/imap-assays#gref.

[55] Inc., PerkinElmer. *AlphaLISA and AlphaScreen No-wash Assays*. 2021 March 23, 2021]; Available from: https://www.perkinelmer.com/lab-products-and-services/application-support-knowledgebase/alphalisa-alphascreen-no-wash-assays/alphalisa-alphascreen-no-washassays-main.html#AlphaLISA AlphaScreenno-washassays-Assayprinciple.

[56] Inc., PerkinElmer. *DELFIA Time-Resolved Fluorescence Assays*. 2021 March 23, 2021]; Available from: https://www.perkinelmer.com/lab-products-and-services/application-support-knowledgebase/delfia/delfia-trf-assays.html#DELFIAtime-resolvedfluo rescenceassays-Assayprinciple.

[57] Scientific, ThermoFisher. *LanthaScreen Kinase Activity Assays*. March 23, 2021]; Available from: https://www.thermofisher.com/il/en/home/industrial/pharma-biopharma/drug-discovery-development/target-and-lead-identification-and-validation/kinasebiology/kinase-activity-assays/lanthascreen-tr-fret-toolbox.html.

[58] Scientific, ThermoFisher. *Adapta® Universal Kinase Assay and Substrates*. March 23, 2021]; Available from: https://www.thermofisher.com/il/en/home/industrial/pharma-biopharma/drug-discovery-development/target-and-lead-identification-and-validation/kinasebiology/kinase-activity-assays/adapta-universal-kinase-assay.html.

[59] Inc., PerkinElmer. *LANCE Ultra Kinase Assays*. 2021 March 23, 2021]; Available from: https://www.perkinelmer.com/lab-products-and-services/application-support-knowledgebase/lance/lance-tr-fret-kinase.html.

[60] Corporation., Promega. *Kinase-Glo® Luminescent Kinase Assays*. 2021 March 23, 2021]; Available from: https://www.promega.com/products/cell-signaling/kinase-assays-and-kinase-biology/kinase_glo-luminescent-kinase-assays/?catNum=V6711.

[61] Nanosyn. *Nanosyn Technology*. 2019 March 23, 2021]; Available from: https://www.nanosyn.com/biology/technology.

[62] Products, Eurofins DiscoverX. *KINOMEscan® Assay Platform*. 2020 March 23, 2021]; Available from: https://www.discoverx.com/technologies-platforms/competitive-binding-technology/kinomescan-technology-platform.

[63] Scientific, ThermoFisher. *LanthaScreen Eu Kinase Binding Assay Technology Overview*. March 23, 2021]; Available from: https://www.thermofisher.com/il/en/home/industrial/pharma-biopharma/drug-discovery-development/target-and-lead-identification-and-validation/kinasebiology/kinase-activity-assays/lanthascreentm-eu-kinase-binding-assay.html.

[64] Fedorov, O., F. H. Niesen, and S. Knapp, *Kinase inhibitor selectivity profiling using differential scanning fluorimetry.* Methods Mol Biol, 2012. **795**: p. 109-118.

[65] Knight, Z. A. and K. M. Shokat, *Features of selective kinase inhibitors.* Chem Biol, 2005. **12**(6): p. 621-637.

[66] Scientific, ThermoFisher. *Z'-LYTE Kinase Assay Kits*. March 23, 2021]; Available from: https://www.thermofisher.com/il/en/home/industrial/pharma-biopharma/drug-discovery-development/target-and-lead-identification-and-validation/kinasebiology/kinase-activity-assays/z-lyte.html.

[67] Dranchak, P., et al., *Profile of the GSK published protein kinase inhibitor set across ATP-dependent and-independent luciferases: implications for reporter-gene assays.* PLoS One, 2013. **8**(3): p. e57888.

[68] Elkins, J. M., et al., *Comprehensive characterization of the Published Kinase Inhibitor Set.* Nat Biotechnol, 2016. **34**(1): p. 95-103.

[69] Davis, M. I., et al., *Comprehensive analysis of kinase inhibitor selectivity.* Nat Biotechnol, 2011. **29**(11): p. 1046-1051.

[70] Karaman, M. W., et al., *A quantitative analysis of kinase inhibitor selectivity.* Nat Biotechnol, 2008. **26**(1): p. 127-132.

[71] Fabian, M. A., et al., *A small molecule-kinase interaction map for clinical kinase inhibitors.* Nat Biotechnol, 2005. **23**(3): p. 329-336.

[72] Fedorov, O., et al., *A systematic interaction map of validated kinase inhibitors with Ser/Thr kinases.* Proc Natl Acad Sci U S A, 2007. **104**(51): p. 20523-20528.

[73] Lo, Y. C., et al., *Computational analysis of kinase inhibitor selectivity using structural knowledge.* Bio informatics, 2019. **35**(2): p. 235-242.

[74] Ferre, F., A. Palmeri, and M. Helmer-Citterich, *Computational methods for analysis and inference of kinase/inhibitor relationships.* Front Genet, 2014. **5**: p. 196.

[75] Pottier, C., et al., *Tyrosine Kinase Inhibitors in Cancer: Breakthrough and Challenges of Targeted Therapy.* Cancers (Basel), 2020. **12**(3).

[76] Uitdehaag, J. C. and G. J. Zaman, *A theoretical entropy score as a single value to express inhibitor selectivity.* BMC Bioinformatics, 2011. **12**: p. 94.

[77] Grant, S. K., *Therapeutic protein kinase inhibitors.* Cell Mol Life Sci, 2009. **66**(7): p. 1163-1177.

[78] Ghoreschi, K., A. Laurence, and J. J. O'Shea, *Selectivity and therapeutic inhibition of kinases: to be or not to be?* Nat Immunol, 2009. **10**(4): p. 356-360.

[79] Villarino, A. V., Y. Kanno, and J. J. O'Shea, *Mechanisms and consequences of Jak-STAT signaling in the immune system.* Nat Immunol, 2017. **18**(4): p. 374-384.

[80] Virtanen, A.T., et al., *Selective JAKinibs: Prospects in Inflammatory and Autoimmune Diseases.* BioDrugs, 2019. **33**(1): p. 15-32.

[81] Wollenhaupt, J., et al., *Safety and efficacy of tofacitinib, an oral janus kinase inhibitor, for the treatment of rheumatoid arthritis in open-label, longterm extension studies.* J Rheumatol, 2014. **41**(5): p. 837-852.

[82] Choy, E. H. S., et al., *The effect of JAK1/JAK2 inhibition in rheumatoid arthritis: efficacy and safety of baricitinib.* Clin Exp Rheumatol, 2019. **37**(4): p. 694-704.

[83] Mesa, R. A., *Ruxolitinib, a selective JAK1 and JAK2 inhibitor for the treatment of myeloproliferative neoplasms and psoriasis.* IDrugs, 2010. **13**(6): p. 394-403.

[84] Mesa, R. A. and J. Cortes, *Optimizing management of ruxolitinib in patients with myelofibrosis: the need for individualized dosing.* J Hematol Oncol, 2013. **6**: p. 79.

[85] Duan, M. and D. Zhou, *Improvement of the hematologic toxicities of ruxolitinib in patients with MPN-associated myelofibrosis using a combination of thalidomide, stanozolol and prednisone.* Hematology, 2019. **24**(1): p. 516-520.

[86] Talpaz, M. and J. J. Kiladjian, *Fedratinib, a newly approved treatment for patients with myeloproliferative neoplasm-associated myelofibrosis.* Leukemia, 2021. **35**(1): p. 1-17.

[87] Bewersdorf, J. P., et al., *Beyond Ruxolitinib: Fedratinib and Other Emergent Treatment Options for Myelofibrosis.* Cancer Manag Res, 2019. **11**: p. 10777-10790.

[88] Ibrahim, F. and D. L. Scott, *Thromboembolism and Janus Kinase Inhibitors.* Drug Saf, 2020. **43**(9): p. 831-833.

[89] Mease, P., et al., *Incidence of venous and arterial thromboembolic events reported in the tofacitinib rheumatoid arthritis, psoriasis and psoriatic arthritis development programmes and from real-world data.* Ann Rheum Dis, 2020. **79**(11): p. 1400-1413.

[90] Kotyla, P. J., et al., *Thromboembolic Adverse Drug Reactions in Janus Kinase (JAK) Inhibitors: Does the Inhibitor*

Specificity Play a Role? Int J Mol Sci, 2021. **22**(5).

[91] Asghar, U., et al., *The history and future of targeting cyclin-dependent kinases in cancer therapy.* Nat Rev Drug Discov, 2015. **14**(2): p. 130-146.

[92] Yuan, K., et al., *Selective inhibition of CDK4/6: A safe and effective strategy for developing anticancer drugs.* Acta Pharm Sin B, 2021. **11**(1): p. 30-54.

[93] O'Leary, B., R. S. Finn, and N. C. Turner, *Treating cancer with selective CDK4/6 inhibitors.* Nat Rev Clin Oncol, 2016. **13**(7): p. 417-430.

[94] Wang, L., et al., *Discovery of a first-in-class CDK2 selective degrader for AML differentiation therapy.* Nat Chem Biol, 2021.

[95] Smidova, V., et al., *Nanomedicine of tyrosine kinase inhibitors.* Theranostics, 2021. **11**(4): p. 1546-1567.

Chapter 3

Using the Structural Kinome to Systematize Kinase Drug Discovery

Zheng Zhao and Philip E. Bourne

Abstract

Kinase-targeted drug design is challenging. It requires designing inhibitors that can bind to specific kinases, when all kinase catalytic domains share a common folding scaffold that binds ATP. Thus, obtaining the desired selectivity, given the whole human kinome, is a fundamental task during early-stage drug discovery. This begins with deciphering the kinase-ligand characteristics, analyzing the structure–activity relationships and prioritizing the desired drug molecules across the whole kinome. Currently, there are more than 300 kinases with released PDB structures, which provides a substantial structural basis to gain these necessary insights. Here, we review *in silico* structure-based methods – notably, a function-site interaction fingerprint approach used in exploring the complete human kinome. *In silico* methods can be explored synergistically with multiple cell-based or protein-based assay platforms such as KINOMEscan. We conclude with new drug discovery opportunities associated with kinase signaling networks and using machine/deep learning techniques broadly referred to as structural biomedical data science.

Keywords: kinase inhibitor, structural kinome, cysteinome, drug design and discovery, drug resistance, protein-ligand interaction fingerprint

1. Introduction

A kinase is an enzyme that catalyzes the transfer of the gamma-phosphate group of ATP to a specific substrate [1, 2]. The human kinome comprises 538 known kinases, and these play an important role in the signal transduction and regulation of cellular functions, such as cell proliferation and necrosis [3, 4]. Correspondingly, dysfunctional kinases are associated with a variety of diseased conditions, such as cancer, inflammatory disease, cardiovascular disease, neurodegenerative disease, and metabolic disease [5, 6]. Therefore, kinases represent important therapeutic targets to overcome these diseases [7] and have become one of the most potentially impactful target families [8–10]. Since the first kinase-targeted drug, imatinib [11], was approved by the US Food and Drug Administration (FDA) in 2001, a significant breakthrough in kinase drug design for cancer treatment [12], 63 small molecule kinase inhibitors have been approved by the FDA [13, 14] as of Feb. 12, 2021. These drugs provide a variety of disease treatments, such as for non-small cell lung cancer (NSCLC) [15], chronic myelogenous leukemia (CML) [16], rheumatoid arthritis [17], breast cancer [18], and acute lymphoblastic leukemia (ALL) [19]. However, in practice, the off-target toxicities and other adverse effects, such as congestive heart failure and cardiogenic shock in some CML patients [20], require the further development of more effective, highly selective inhibitors [3].

Attaining such high selectivity is a daunting task since the inhibitor should bind to a specific primary kinase or selected kinases, yet all kinase catalytic domains share a common folding scaffold that binds ATP [21]. To validate selectivity, kinome-scale screening of lead compounds has been attracting more attention [22, 23]. Indeed, there are a number of experimental kinome-scale screening methods [22, 24], such as KinaseProfiler [25], KINOMEscan [26], and KiNativ [27]. Although kinase profiling technologies are gradually maturing, they are expensive, especially for screening a large compound library against the whole kinome, which remains impractical.

With the availability of an increasing number of kinase structures, virtual structure-based drug screening provides a low-cost and effective way to filter a large compound library and identify the most likely compounds at an early stage of drug screening. Used concurrently with experiential profiling platforms, in silico methods provide early-stage kinome-scale drug screening. Based on structural insights, the atom-level binding characteristics of every compound can be revealed and can be used as a guideline for further compound identification and optimization. Given the more than 300 kinases with released PDB structures, subtle differences have been found in the vicinity of the binding site where the adenine base of ATP binds, as well as binding sites away from the ATP binding site, such as in the C lobe of the kinase domain [28, 29]. This structural corpora provides insights toward achieving the desired selectivity.

In this chapter we describe the characterization of the whole structure kinome to facilitate drug development. Specifically, we use the function-site fingerprint method to analyze the structural kinome providing systematic insights into kinase drug discovery. With increased knowledge of kinase-driven signaling pathways new kinase targets are continuously being explored for related disease treatment. Looking ahead to structural biomedical data science, combining structure-based polypharmacology with machine/deep learning new challenges and opportunities are discussed.

2. Kinome-level profiling

Due to the common ATP-binding pocket, the kinase domain was thought to be undruggable prior to the 1990s [30]. With advances in protein- and cell-level experimental techniques and an increase in structure-based knowledge of protein kinases, variation among different kinases became apparent [31]. However, possible specificity requires kinome-scale validation. Moreover, with the increased knowledge of kinase signal pathways, traditional "one-drug-one-target" models have been replaced by the acceptance of polypharmacology. Examples include the FDA-approved drug Crizotinib targeting ALK and Met for treating NSCLC, and Cabozantinib targeting VEGFR, MET, RET, FLT1/3/4, AXL, and TIE2 for treating thyroid cancer. Hence, kinome-level profiling is an important step in confirming the selectivity of multi-target drugs.

Multiple commercial platforms provide kinome profiling services with panels ranging from 30 to 715 kinases (**Table 1**) [1, 32, 33].

Apart from revealing off-targets, profiling inhibitors offers new opportunities for drug discovery [23, 34–39]. Through profiling, the target spectrum reveals the compound's selectivity based on the coverage of kinases it hits, including unexpected off-target interactions, which is a cost-effective way of jumpstarting new kinase drug discovery [40]. For example, Druker et al. utilized an *in vitro* profiling panel of 30 kinases to establish the selectivity of imatinib in 1996 [16]. Later scientists revisited the successful drug using a larger profiling panel and found that

Providers	Technologies	Kinases	Results	Websites
Reaction biology	HotSpot™ ^{33}PanQinase™	715	IC_{50}	https://www.reactionbiology.com
DiscoverRx	KinomeScan	489	Kd/ IC_{50}	https://www.discoverx.com
Thermo Fisher Scientific	Z′-LYTE Adapta	>485	IC_{50}/ EC50	https://www.thermofisher.com
Eurofins Discovery	KinaseProfiler™	>420	IC_{50}	https://www.eurofinsdiscoveryservices.com
Luceome Biotechnologies	KinaseSeeker™ KinaseLite™	409	IC_{50}	https://www.luceome.com
ActivX Biosciences	KiNativ™	>400	Kd/ IC_{50}	https://www.kinativ.com

Table 1.
Commercial kinase profiling service providers as of Feb. 28, 2021, based on the provider's webpages.

imatinib has multiple off-targets in the human kinome. By utilizing the off-target interactions, imatinib can be repurposed for other diseases. Indeed, in 2008 the FDA approved imatinib as an adjuvant treatment to CD117-positive gastrointestinal stromal tumors (GIST) in adult patients [41, 42].

3. Structural kinome

Profiling the whole human kinome as a routine procedure can validate the selectivity of any given compound by comparing the binding affinities, such as IC_{50} or Kd [10, 43]. Subsequently optimizing the compound toward the desired selectivity is the next critical step in early-stage drug discovery. This often begins with deciphering the kinase-ligand characteristics and analyzing the structure–activity relationships, such as confirming which part of the binding sites is nucleophilic/electrophilic, which sub-pocket is hydrophobic, or which amino acids can provide covalent interactions. These atom-level interaction details provide the basic principles by which to modify the functional groups of the given compound. Iteratively combining compound optimization with kinome profiling establishes lead compounds for further testing.

As of Feb. 2021, there are 304 kinases associated with 5208 PDB structures covering all kinase groups, i.e., AGC (276 structures), Atypical (255 structures), CAMK (587 structures), CK1 (82 structures), CMGC (1428 structures), STE (296 structures), TK (1447 structures), TKL (335 structures), and other (493 structures) [44, 45]. The 3-D kinase structure corpus provides a basis for structural kinome-based drug discovery. Scientists can not only directly review the compound binding details against the specific target, but they can also compare nuances -similarities and differences - among different kinase targets. For example, in comparing the ATP binding mode, 63 FDA-approved small-molecule kinase drugs can be divided into Type-I, II, III, or IV inhibitors [29, 46]. Similarly, based on the possible existence of a covalent interactions, these kinase drugs can be divided into covalent (irreversible) inhibitors and noncovalent (reversible) inhibitors (**Table 2**) [47, 48]. Overall, the desired selectivity is achieved by utilizing every nuance of the different binding sites and accommodating the different sub-pockets of the binding sites among the different kinases [13, 46, 49]. As such, deciphering the whole structural kinome will be very useful in enhancing kinase inhibitor screening, optimization, and prediction. To this end, we introduce the alignment of the binding sites across the structural kinome and describe the characteristics of the aligned binding sites for achieving the desired selectivity.

Drug	Type	Mode	PDB ID	Drug	Type	Mode	PDB ID
Imatinib	II	Reversible	1OPJ	Brigatinib	I	Reversible	5J7H
Gefitinib	I	Reversible	4I22	Midostaurin	I	Reversible	4NCT
Erlotinib	I	Reversible	4HJO	Neratinib	I	Irreversible	2JIV
Sorafenib	II	Reversible	4ASD	Abemaciclib	I	Reversible	5L2S
Sunitinib	I	Reversible	2Y7J	Copanlisib	I	Reversible	5G2N
Dasatinib	I	Reversible	3QLG	Acalabrutinib	I	Irreversible	—
Lapatinib	I	Reversible	1XKK	Netarsudil	I	Reversible	—
Nilotinib	II	Reversible	3GP0	Fostamatinib	I	Reversible	3FQS
Pazopanib	I	Reversible	—	Baricitinib	I	Reversible	4W9X
Vandetanib	I	Reversible	2IVU	Binimetinib	III	Reversible	6V2X
Crizotinib	I	Reversible	3ZBF	Encorafenib	I	Reversible	—
Vemurafenib	I	Reversible	3OG7	Dacomitinib	I	Irreversible	4I24
Ruxolitinib	I	Reversible	4U5J	Gilteritinib	I	Reversible	7AB1
Axitinib	I	Reversible	4AGC	Larotrectinib	I	Reversible	—
Bosutinib	I	Reversible	4OTW	Lorlatinib	I	Reversible	5A9U
Regorafenib	II	Reversible	—	Entrectinib	I	Reversible	5FTO
Tofacitinib	I	Reversible	3LXN	Erdafitinib	I	Reversible	5EW8
Cabozantinib	II	Reversible	—	Fedratinib	I	Reversible	6VNE
Ponatinib	II	Reversible	4C8B	Pexidartinib	II	Reversible	4R7H
Trametinib	III	Reversible	7JUR	Upadacitinib	I	Reversible	—
Dabrafenib	I	Reversible	4XV2	Zanubrutinib	I	Irreversible	6J6M
Afatinib	I	Irreversible	4G5J	Pemigatinib	I	Rreversible	—
Ibrutinib	I	Irreversible	5P9I	Pralsetinib	I	Rreversible	7JU5
Ceritinib	I	Reversible	4MKC	Ripretinib	II	Reversible	6MOB
Idelalisib	I	Reversible	4XE0	Selpercatinib	I	Rreversible	7JU6
Nintedanib	I	Reversible	3C7Q	Selumetinib	III	Reversible	4U7Z
Palbociclib	I	Reversible	2EUF	Tucatinib	I	Rreversible	—
Lenvatinib	I	Reversible	3WZD	Avapritinib	I	Rreversible	—
Cobimetinib	III	Reversible	4AN2	Capmatinib	I	Rreversible	5EOB
Osimertinib	I	Irreversible	4ZAU	Tepotinib	I	Rreversible	4R1V
Alectinib	I	Reversible	5XV7	Trilaciclib	I	Rreversible	—
Ribociclib	I	Reversible	5L2T				

Table 2.
63 FDA-approved kinase small molecule drugs as of Feb. 12, 2021. Columns 2–4 show that the inhibitor types (column 2), covalent interaction modes (column 3), and PDB IDs if the drug-bound structure is available in the PDB (column 4; "-" means the drug-bound PDB structure is unavailable).

Zhao et al. developed a function-site interaction fingerprint (FsIFP) approach to align and delineate the structural human kinome [29]. The FsIFP approach describes protein–ligand interaction characteristics at the functional site using 1D fingerprints [50], which can be compared and contrasted. The approach consists of three steps (**Figure 1**). First, preparing the structural kinome database. All the released PDB structures can be directly downloaded based on keyword search or the kinase enzyme index [44]. Additionally, there are a few kinase-specific webpages such as UniProt (https://www.uniprot.org/docs/pkinfam), KLIFS [45] (https://klifs.net/), and the kinase sarfari https://chembl.gitbook.io/chembl-interface-documentation/legacy-resources#kinase-sarfari). Second, aligning the binding sites. The SMAP software [51], one sequence-independent binding site comparison tool, was applied to compare all of the binding sites. Third, encoding the interaction fingerprint. Given any protein-ligand complex, every involved residue comprising the functional site is converted into a fingerprint string by using the predefined standards [52] for different residue-ligand nonbinding interactions such as van der Waals, aromatic stacking interactions, hydrogen-bond interactions, and electrostatic interactions [53]. Currently, there are a few open-source tools available, such as IChem [54] and PyPlif [55] that provide these data. The function-site interaction fingerprints are obtained by combining the aligned binding sites with

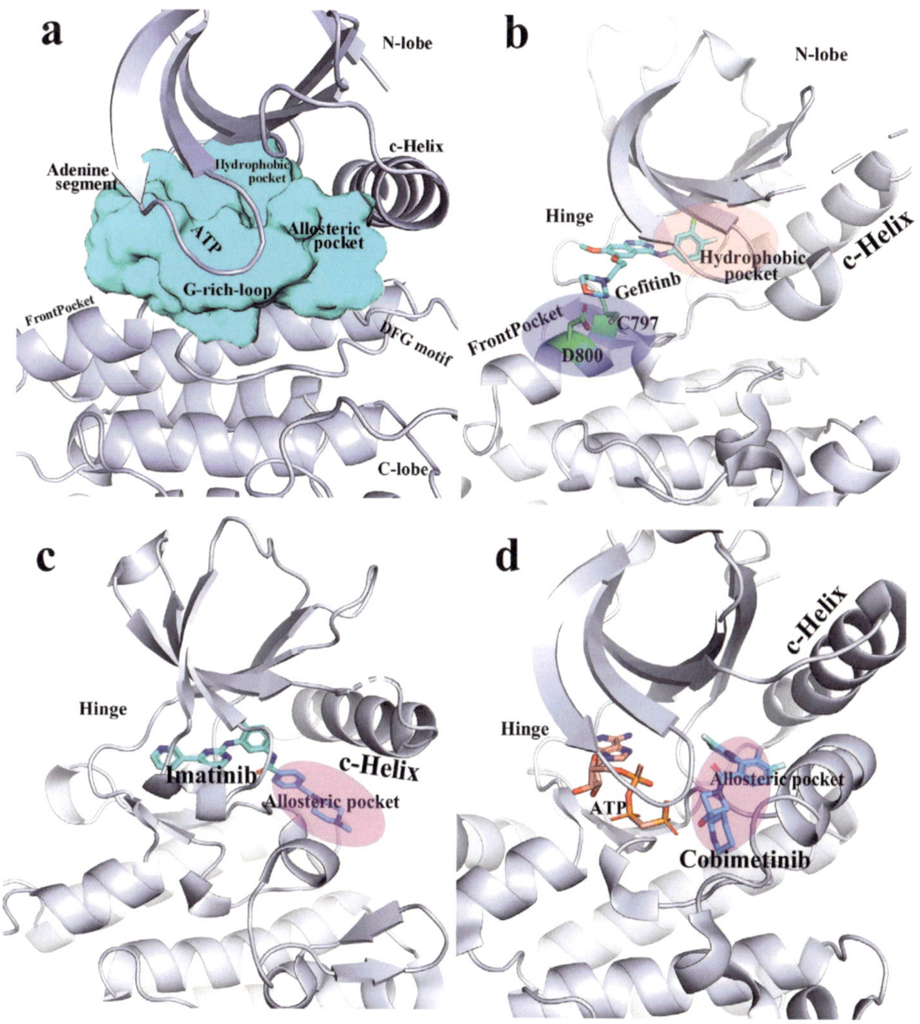

Figure 1.
(a) Kinase binding site surrounding the ATP binding cavity (PDB ID: 1 m17 as the template). (b). The occupied binding pocket of a type-I kinase inhibitor (PDB ID: 4i22). (c) the binding characteristics of a type-II kinase inhibitor (PDB ID: 2hyy); (d) the binding characteristics of a type-III kinase inhibitor (PDB ID: 4an2).

the encoded interaction fingerprints. So far, the FsIFP strategy has been successfully applied to a number of different drug design and discovery projects [15, 56–58].

The FsIFP approach, which examines the specificity among binding sites has been explored to design high-selectivity kinase inhibitors. Beyond the ATP binding pocket, there are other binding subpockets to be validated [59], such as hydrophobic segment, allosteric segment, DFG motif area, and G-rich-loop region (**Figure 1a**). Corresponding to these binding regions, inhibitors are classified as Type-I, Type-II, and Type-III.

Type-I kinase inhibitors mainly bind to the ATP-binding site in the "DFG-in" conformation. To obtain stronger binding affinity and greater selectivity than ATP, besides occupying the ATP-binding space, Type-I inhibitors extend into different proximal regions, specifically referred to as the front pocket region, the hydrophobic pocket region, the DFG motif, or the G-rich-loop region [13, 59]. For example, Gefitinib is one Type-I drug for the treatment of non-small cell lung cancer (NSCLC) [60]. Its quinazoline scaffold forms hydrogen bonds with the hinge region like the adenine moiety of ATP (**Figure 1b**). More importantly, the 3-chloro-4-fluorophenyl fragment of Gefitinib extends into the hydrophobic pocket, and the morpholine derivative binds at the front pocket and forms polar interactions with residues Cys797 and Asp800 (**Figure 1b**) [61]. In contrast, Type-II kinase inhibitor typically bind in the "DFG-out" conformation. Type-II kinase inhibitors extend into the allosteric pocket region beyond the ATP binding pocket. For example, Imatinib is a Type-II inhibitor to treat positive acute lymphoblastic leukemia (Ph + ALL) in children. Like Type-I inhibitors, there is a scaffold fragment (**Figure 1c**) occupying the space where the adenine moity of ATP binds. At the same time, the 4-(4-Methyl-piperazin-1-ylmethyl) benzamide extends into the allosteric pocket. Type-III inhibitors occupy the allosteric pocket (**Figure 1d**), which is not so well conserved that attractive for designing non-ATP competitive kinase inhibitors. Fingerprints established through aligned structures provide detailed information on the binding sites occupied by Type- I, II, and III kinase inhibitors.

The other noteworthy aspect is the difference in amino acids at the same spatial position among the aligned binding sites, which is useful in obtaining the desired selectivity. Typically, structural kinome-guided studies have shown that there are a number of cysteine residues distributed around the binding sites [1, 21, 62, 63]. In Zhang et al.'s review, they identified over 200 kinases bearing at least one cysteine

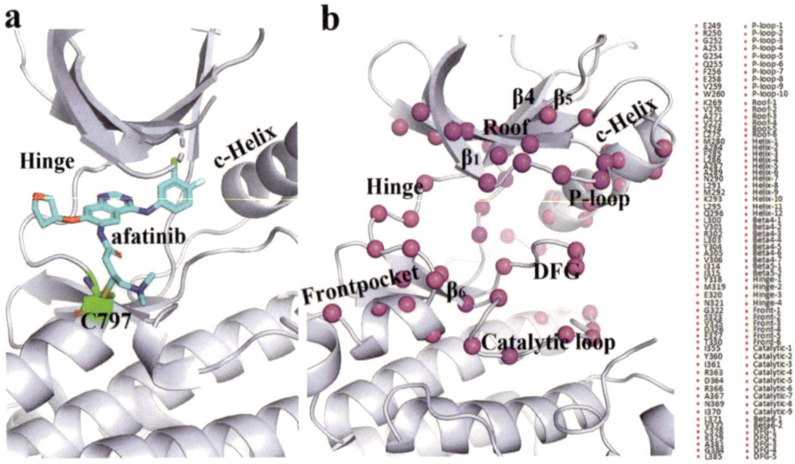

Figure 2.
(a) Covalent binding mode of Afatinib (PDB id: 4g5j). (b) 63 positions bearing the accessible cysteines (PDB id: 3byu). The legend shows the amino acids and the corresponding spatial positions (purple balls).

in and around the ATP binding pocket, thus highlighting the broad structural basis to improve the selectivity and binding affinity by covalently utilizing these non-catalytic cysteines [21]. Currently, 7 covalent kinase inhibitors have been approved (**Table 2**). This class of inhibitors not only bind to the ATP binding pocket, but also hit nearby cysteine to form covalent interaction; Afatinib (**Figure 2a**) being one example through binding to Cys797. Similarly, the other 6 inhibitors all form covalent bonds with the corresponding cysteines located in the front pocket. Like Afatinib, Osimertinib, Dacomitinib, and Neratinib all have covalent interaction with Cys797 in the EGFR crystal structure (**Figure 2a**). Ibrutinib, Acalabrutinib, and Zanubrutinib all form covalent interactions with Cys481, targeting BTK. In their study, Zhao et al [63] identified 63 different amino acid locations bearing accessible cysteines through surveying the whole structural kinome (**Figure 2b**), speaking to the broad applicability of designing covalent kinase inhibitors.

4. Challenges and opportunities

Since the launch of the first kinase drug, Imatinib in 2001, kinase targeted drug discovery has been on a fast track. In the last six years, an average of eight small molecule kinase drugs have been approved per year. This tremendous success benefits patients, but also highlights our ability to achieve drug discovery outcomes [9, 64]. However, challenges still remain in the development of efficient, non-toxic kinase-targeted drugs [3].

Clinical adverse effects are one major challenge. For example, kinase drugs affect the digestive system and cause nausea, vomiting, and/or diarrhoea [65]. Further, most kinase inhibitors cause serious adverse effects, such as different degrees of cytopenia [66]. These side effects typically result from off-targets effects. To avoid such side effects, a highly selective drug is desired. Alternatively, adverse effect can be due to on-target toxicities involving the intrinsic mechanisms of the drugs [67]. At this point in the evolution of small molecule kinase drugs, novel compound scaffolds are needed to reduce adverse effect as much as possible. Maximizing the diversity of molecular scaffolds is critically important for extracting the novel compound early on. The increasing availability of panels of phenotypic assays may provide one strategy to profile selectivity by combining virtual structure-based kinome screening, which can filter a huge compound library into a highly focused kinase library [68].

Another challenge is acquired drug resistance [58, 69]. In clinical practice, kinase-targeted drugs are frequently subject to drug resistance, which has become a primary vulnerability in targeted cancer therapy. The first difficulty is exploring resistance mechanisms due to the diversity of specific drug-binding mechanisms. For example, drug resistance of Erlotinib, which is one FDA-approved kinase drug used to treat patients with EGFR-overexpression induced NSCLC, is caused by the gatekeeper T790M mutation, which increases the binding affinity of ATP to the EGFR kinase [70]. In another example, Crizotinib was often found to be ineffective in the majority of patients after 1–2 years' treatment against ALK-positive NSCLC due to the acquired ALK L1196M mutation, which decreased the binding affinity of Crizotinib [71].

Nevertheless, these challenges also provide unique opportunities to develop new approaches and applications. Currently, in vitro and/or in vivo kinome-scale and proteome-scale profiling methodologies have been merged into the drug design pipeline, which potentially provides a thorough understanding of targets and selectivity of kinase inhibitors. Combined with the diseases' signal pathway, the target spectrum can be further applied to "one-drug-multiple-target" drug design. For example, Midostaurin is a multi-target kinase drug [72] used to treat adult

Provider	Technology	Coverage	Resource website
Reaction biology	HotSpot™	300 Kinases × 178 Inhibitors	www.guidetopharmacology.org
ChEMBL Kinase SARfari	Collected from academic publications	~530,000 data points	www.ebi.ac.uk/chembl
Eurofins Discovery	KinaseProfiler™	234 Kinases × 158 Inhibitors	www.guidetopharmacology.org
DiscoverRx	KinomeScan	~440 Kinases × 182 Inhibitors	lincs.hms.harvard.edu
ActivX Biosciences	KiNativ™	(194 to 316) Kinases × 30 Inhibitors	lincs.hms.harvard.edu

Table 3.
Kinase-inhibitor interaction activity data resource.

patients with newly diagnosed FLT3-mutated acute myeloid leukemia (AML). For a "multiple-drug-multiple-target" combination therapy strategy, Capmatinib (a MET inhibitor) and Gefitinib (an EGFR inhibitor) had been approved to treat patients with EGFR-mutated-MET-dysregulated – in particular, MET-amplified - NSCLC [73]. We can expect profiling methodologies will be further developed to cover the whole kinome and even the proteome.

In virtual drug design and discovery, the incorporation of machine/deep learning and structural biomedical data science are advancing compound screening, target validation, and selectivity improvement [74]. Currently, data science has become one of the fastest-growing disciplines and deep learning has been applied to drug synthesis, design, and prediction [75–77]. Moreover, there are a large number of kinase assay databases available. For example, a database from Merck, KGaA, with over 1.0 million data points (i.e., 4,712 compounds x 220 kinases). Merget et al. used it to train one virtual profiling assay model to support virtual screening, compound repurposing, and the detection of potential off-targets [37]. Here, we collate the free databases of available kinase-inhibitor activity (**Table 3**). It is worth noting that the ChEMBL Kinase SARfari database, which contains ~54,000 compounds, ~980 kinases targets, and the corresponding approximately 530 K structure–activity data points [78], has been used to predict kinome-wide profiling of small molecules [79–81]. Taken together, data-driven methods and applications will further experimental protocols and facilitate the drug discovery processes.

Author details

Zheng Zhao and Philip E. Bourne*
Department of Biomedical Engineering, School of Data Science, University of Virginia, Charlottesville, Virginia, United States of America

*Address all correspondence to: peb6a@virginia.edu

References

[1] Liu, Q.; Sabnis, Y.; Zhao, Z.; Zhang, T.; Buhrlage, S. J.; Jones, L. H.; Gray, N. S., Developing irreversible inhibitors of the protein kinase cysteinome. Chem Biol **2013,** *20* (2), 146-159.

[2] Fleuren, E. D.; Zhang, L.; Wu, J.; Daly, R. J., The kinome 'at large' in cancer. Nat Rev Cancer **2016,** *16* (2), 83-98.

[3] Gharwan, H.; Groninger, H., Kinase inhibitors and monoclonal antibodies in oncology: clinical implications. Nat Rev Clin Oncol **2016,** *13* (4), 209-227.

[4] Santos, R.; Ursu, O.; Gaulton, A.; Bento, A. P.; Donadi, R. S.; Bologa, C. G.; Karlsson, A.; Al-Lazikani, B.; Hersey, A.; Oprea, T. I.; Overington, J. P., A comprehensive map of molecular drug targets. Nat Rev Drug Discov **2017,** *16* (1), 19-34.

[5] Lahiry, P.; Torkamani, A.; Schork, N. J.; Hegele, R. A., Kinase mutations in human disease: interpreting genotype-phenotype relationships. Nat Rev Genet **2010,** *11* (1), 60-74.

[6] Vogelstein, B.; Papadopoulos, N.; Velculescu, V. E.; Zhou, S.; Diaz, L. A., Jr.; Kinzler, K. W., Cancer genome landscapes. Science **2013,** *339* (6127), 1546-1558.

[7] Bhullar, K. S.; Lagaron, N. O.; McGowan, E. M.; Parmar, I.; Jha, A.; Hubbard, B. P.; Rupasinghe, H. P. V., Kinase-targeted cancer therapies: progress, challenges and future directions. Mol Cancer **2018,** *17* (1), 48.

[8] Fabbro, D., 25 years of small molecular weight kinase inhibitors: potentials and limitations. Mol Pharmacol **2015,** *87* (5), 766-775.

[9] Ferguson, F. M.; Gray, N. S., Kinase inhibitors: the road ahead. Nat Rev Drug Discov **2018,** *17* (5), 353-377.

[10] Wilson, L. J.; Linley, A.; Hammond, D. E.; Hood, F. E.; Coulson, J. M.; MacEwan, D. J.; Ross, S. J.; Slupsky, J. R.; Smith, P. D.; Eyers, P. A.; Prior, I. A., New Perspectives, Opportunities, and Challenges in Exploring the Human Protein Kinome. Cancer Res **2018,** *78* (1), 15-29.

[11] Druker, B. J.; Talpaz, M.; Resta, D. J.; Peng, B.; Buchdunger, E.; Ford, J. M.; Lydon, N. B.; Kantarjian, H.; Capdeville, R.; Ohno-Jones, S.; Sawyers, C. L., Efficacy and safety of a specific inhibitor of the BCR-ABL tyrosine kinase in chronic myeloid leukemia. N Engl J Med **2001,** *344* (14), 1031-1037.

[12] Druker, B. J.; Guilhot, F.; O'Brien, S. G.; Gathmann, I.; Kantarjian, H.; Gattermann, N.; Deininger, M. W.; Silver, R. T.; Goldman, J. M.; Stone, R. M.; Cervantes, F.; Hochhaus, A.; Powell, B. L.; Gabrilove, J. L.; Rousselot, P.; Reiffers, J.; Cornelissen, J. J.; Hughes, T.; Agis, H.; Fischer, T.; Verhoef, G.; Shepherd, J.; Saglio, G.; Gratwohl, A.; Nielsen, J. L.; Radich, J. P.; Simonsson, B.; Taylor, K.; Baccarani, M.; So, C.; Letvak, L.; Larson, R. A.; Investigators, I., Five-year follow-up of patients receiving imatinib for chronic myeloid leukemia. *N Engl J Med* **2006,** *355* (23), 2408-17.

[13] Zhao, Z.; Bourne, P. E., Overview of Current Type I/II Kinase Inhibitors. In *Next Generation Kinase Inhibitors*, 2020; pp 13-28.

[14] Roskoski, R., Jr., Properties of FDA-approved small molecule protein kinase inhibitors: A 2020 update. Pharmacol Res **2020,** *152*, 104609.

[15] Zhao, Z.; Xie, L.; Bourne, P. E., Structural Insights into Characterizing Binding Sites in Epidermal Growth Factor Receptor Kinase Mutants. J Chem Inf Model **2019,** *59* (1), 453-462.

[16] Druker, B. J.; Tamura, S.; Buchdunger, E.; Ohno, S.; Segal, G. M.; Fanning, S.; Zimmermann, J.; Lydon, N. B., Effects of a selective inhibitor of the Abl tyrosine kinase on the growth of Bcr-Abl positive cells. Nat Med **1996,** *2* (5), 561-566.

[17] Harrington, R.; Al Nokhatha, S. A.; Conway, R., JAK Inhibitors in Rheumatoid Arthritis: An Evidence-Based Review on the Emerging Clinical Data. J Inflamm Res **2020,** *13*, 519-531.

[18] Wilcock, P.; Webster, R. M., The breast cancer drug market. *Nat Rev Drug Discov* **2021**.

[19] Hirschbuhl, K.; Labopin, M.; Houhou, M.; Gabellier, L.; Labussiere-Wallet, H.; Lioure, B.; Beelen, D.; Cornelissen, J.; Wulf, G.; Jindra, P.; Tilly, H.; Passweg, J.; Niittyvuopio, R.; Bug, G.; Schmid, C.; Nagler, A.; Giebel, S.; Mohty, M., Second- and third-generation tyrosine kinase inhibitors for Philadelphia-positive adult acute lymphoblastic leukemia relapsing post allogeneic stem cell transplantation-a registry study on behalf of the EBMT Acute Leukemia Working Party. *Bone Marrow Transplant* **2020**.

[20] Food and Drug Administration. Gleevec (imatinib): full prescribing information. Drugs@FDA, https://www.accessdata.fda.gov/drugsatfda_docs/label/2014/021588s040lbl.pdf. 2014.

[21] Zhang, J.; Yang, P. L.; Gray, N. S., Targeting cancer with small molecule kinase inhibitors. Nat Rev Cancer **2009,** *9* (1), 28-39.

[22] Wang, Y.; Ma, H., Protein kinase profiling assays: a technology review. Drug Discov Today Technol **2015,** *18*, 1-8.

[23] Klaeger, S.; Heinzlmeir, S.; Wilhelm, M.; Polzer, H.; Vick, B.; Koenig, P. A.; Reinecke, M.; Ruprecht, B.; Petzoldt, S.; Meng, C.; Zecha, J.; Reiter, K.; Qiao, H.; Helm, D.; Koch, H.; Schoof, M.; Canevari, G.; Casale, E.; Depaolini, S. R.; Feuchtinger, A.; Wu, Z.; Schmidt, T.; Rueckert, L.; Becker, W.; Huenges, J.; Garz, A. K.; Gohlke, B. O.; Zolg, D. P.; Kayser, G.; Vooder, T.; Preissner, R.; Hahne, H.; Tonisson, N.; Kramer, K.; Gotze, K.; Bassermann, F.; Schlegl, J.; Ehrlich, H. C.; Aiche, S.; Walch, A.; Greif, P. A.; Schneider, S.; Felder, E. R.; Ruland, J.; Medard, G.; Jeremias, I.; Spiekermann, K.; Kuster, B., The target landscape of clinical kinase drugs. *Science* **2017,** *358* (6367).

[24] Wu, P.; Givskov, M.; Nielsen, T. E., Kinase Inhibitors. In *Drug Selectivity: An Evolving Concept in Medicinal Chemistry*, Handler, N.; Buschmann, H.; Mannhold, R.; Holenz, J., Eds. Wiley: 2017; pp 33-53.

[25] Gao, Y.; Davies, S. P.; Augustin, M.; Woodward, A.; Patel, U. A.; Kovelman, R.; Harvey, K. J., A broad activity screen in support of a chemogenomic map for kinase signalling research and drug discovery. Biochem J **2013,** *451* (2), 313-328.

[26] Karaman, M. W.; Herrgard, S.; Treiber, D. K.; Gallant, P.; Atteridge, C. E.; Campbell, B. T.; Chan, K. W.; Ciceri, P.; Davis, M. I.; Edeen, P. T.; Faraoni, R.; Floyd, M.; Hunt, J. P.; Lockhart, D. J.; Milanov, Z. V.; Morrison, M. J.; Pallares, G.; Patel, H. K.; Pritchard, S.; Wodicka, L. M.; Zarrinkar, P. P., A quantitative analysis of kinase inhibitor selectivity. Nat Biotechnol **2008,** *26* (1), 127-132.

[27] Patricelli, M. P.; Szardenings, A. K.; Liyanage, M.; Nomanbhoy, T. K.; Wu, M.; Weissig, H.; Aban, A.; Chun, D.; Tanner, S.; Kozarich, J. W., Functional interrogation of the kinome using nucleotide acyl phosphates. Biochemistry **2007,** *46* (2), 350-358.

[28] Muller, S.; Chaikuad, A.; Gray, N. S.; Knapp, S., The ins and outs of

selective kinase inhibitor development. Nat Chem Biol **2015,** *11* (11), 818-821.

[29] Zhao, Z.; Xie, L.; Xie, L.; Bourne, P. E., Delineation of Polypharmacology across the Human Structural Kinome Using a Functional Site Interaction Fingerprint Approach. J Med Chem **2016,** *59* (9), 4326-4341.

[30] Crews, C. M., Targeting the undruggable proteome: the small molecules of my dreams. Chem Biol **2010,** *17* (6), 551-555.

[31] Dang, C. V.; Reddy, E. P.; Shokat, K. M.; Soucek, L., Drugging the 'undruggable' cancer targets. Nat Rev Cancer **2017,** *17* (8), 502-508.

[32] Bamborough, P., System-based drug discovery within the human kinome. Expert Opin Drug Discov **2012,** *7* (11), 1053-1070.

[33] Wu, P.; Givskov, M.; Nielsen, T. E., Kinase Inhibitors. In *Drug Selectivity*, 2017; pp 31-53.

[34] Bamborough, P.; Drewry, D.; Harper, G.; Smith, G. K.; Schneider, K., Assessment of chemical coverage of kinome space and its implications for kinase drug discovery. J Med Chem **2008,** *51* (24), 7898-7914.

[35] Sutherland, J. J.; Gao, C.; Cahya, S.; Vieth, M., What general conclusions can we draw from kinase profiling data sets? Biochim Biophys Acta **2013,** *1834* (7), 1425-1433.

[36] Jacoby, E.; Tresadern, G.; Bembenek, S.; Wroblowski, B.; Buyck, C.; Neefs, J. M.; Rassokhin, D.; Poncelet, A.; Hunt, J.; van Vlijmen, H., Extending kinome coverage by analysis of kinase inhibitor broad profiling data. Drug Discov Today **2015,** *20* (6), 652-658.

[37] Merget, B.; Turk, S.; Eid, S.; Rippmann, F.; Fulle, S., Profiling Prediction of Kinase Inhibitors: Toward the Virtual Assay. J Med Chem **2017,** *60* (1), 474-485.

[38] Bembenek, S. D.; Hirst, G.; Mirzadegan, T., Determination of a Focused Mini Kinase Panel for Early Identification of Selective Kinase Inhibitors. J Chem Inf Model **2018,** *58* (7), 1434-1440.

[39] Wells, C. I.; Al-Ali, H.; Andrews, D. M.; Asquith, C. R. M.; Axtman, A. D.; Dikic, I.; Ebner, D.; Ettmayer, P.; Fischer, C.; Frederiksen, M.; Futrell, R. E.; Gray, N. S.; Hatch, S. B.; Knapp, S.; Lucking, U.; Michaelides, M.; Mills, C. E.; Muller, S.; Owen, D.; Picado, A.; Saikatendu, K. S.; Schroder, M.; Stolz, A.; Tellechea, M.; Turunen, B. J.; Vilar, S.; Wang, J.; Zuercher, W. J.; Willson, T. M.; Drewry, D. H., The Kinase Chemogenomic Set (KCGS): An Open Science Resource for Kinase Vulnerability Identification. *Int J Mol Sci* **2021,** *22* (2).

[40] Goldstein, D. M.; Gray, N. S.; Zarrinkar, P. P., High-throughput kinase profiling as a platform for drug discovery. Nat Rev Drug Discov **2008,** *7* (5), 391-397.

[41] Su, E. J.; Fredriksson, L.; Geyer, M.; Folestad, E.; Cale, J.; Andrae, J.; Gao, Y.; Pietras, K.; Mann, K.; Yepes, M.; Strickland, D. K.; Betsholtz, C.; Eriksson, U.; Lawrence, D. A., Activation of PDGF-CC by tissue plasminogen activator impairs blood-brain barrier integrity during ischemic stroke. Nat Med **2008,** *14* (7), 731-737.

[42] Lopes, L. F.; Bacchi, C. E., Imatinib treatment for gastrointestinal stromal tumour (GIST). J Cell Mol Med **2010,** *14* (1-2), 42-50.

[43] Miduturu, C. V.; Deng, X.; Kwiatkowski, N.; Yang, W.; Brault, L.; Filippakopoulos, P.; Chung, E.; Yang, Q.; Schwaller, J.; Knapp, S.; King, R. W.; Lee, J. D.; Herrgard, S.; Zarrinkar, P.; Gray, N. S., High-throughput kinase

profiling: a more efficient approach toward the discovery of new kinase inhibitors. Chem Biol **2011,** *18* (7), 868-879.

[44] Berman, H. M.; Westbrook, J.; Feng, Z.; Gilliland, G.; Bhat, T. N.; Weissig, H.; Shindyalov, I. N.; Bourne, P. E., The Protein Data Bank. Nucleic Acids Res **2000,** *28* (1), 235-242.

[45] Kanev, G. K.; de Graaf, C.; Westerman, B. A.; de Esch, I. J. P.; Kooistra, A. J., KLIFS: an overhaul after the first 5 years of supporting kinase research. Nucleic Acids Res **2021,** *49* (D1), D562-D569.

[46] Roskoski, R., Jr., Classification of small molecule protein kinase inhibitors based upon the structures of their drug-enzyme complexes. Pharmacol Res **2016,** *103*, 26-48.

[47] Zhao, Z.; Bourne, P. E., Progress with covalent small-molecule kinase inhibitors. Drug Discov Today **2018,** *23* (3), 727-735.

[48] Lu, W.; Kostic, M.; Zhang, T.; Che, J.; Patricelli, M. P.; Jones, L. H.; Chouchani, E. T.; Gray, N. S., Fragment-based covalent ligand discovery. RSC Chemical Biology **2021**.

[49] Zhao, Z.; Wu, H.; Wang, L.; Liu, Y.; Knapp, S.; Liu, Q.; Gray, N. S., Exploration of type II binding mode: A privileged approach for kinase inhibitor focused drug discovery? ACS Chem Biol **2014,** *9* (6), 1230-1241.

[50] Deng, Z.; Chuaqui, C.; Singh, J., Structural interaction fingerprint (SIFt): a novel method for analyzing three-dimensional protein-ligand binding interactions. J Med Chem **2004,** *47* (2), 337-344.

[51] Xie, L.; Bourne, P. E., A robust and efficient algorithm for the shape description of protein structures and its application in predicting ligand binding sites. *BMC Bioinformatics* **2007,** *8 Suppl 4*, S9.

[52] Kellenberger, E.; Muller, P.; Schalon, C.; Bret, G.; Foata, N.; Rognan, D., sc-PDB: an annotated database of druggable binding sites from the Protein Data Bank. J Chem Inf Model **2006,** *46* (2), 717-727.

[53] Marcou, G.; Rognan, D., Optimizing fragment and scaffold docking by use of molecular interaction fingerprints. J Chem Inf Model **2007,** *47* (1), 195-207.

[54] Desaphy, J.; Raimbaud, E.; Ducrot, P.; Rognan, D., Encoding protein-ligand interaction patterns in fingerprints and graphs. J Chem Inf Model **2013,** *53* (3), 623-637.

[55] Radifar, M.; Yuniarti, N.; Istyastono, E. P., PyPLIF: Python-based Protein-Ligand Interaction Fingerprinting. Bioinformation **2013,** *9* (6), 325-328.

[56] Zhao, Z.; Xie, L.; Bourne, P. E., Insights into the binding mode of MEK type-III inhibitors. A step towards discovering and designing allosteric kinase inhibitors across the human kinome. *PLoS One* **2017,** *12* (6), e0179936.

[57] Zhao, Z.; Bourne, P. E., Structural Insights into the Binding Modes of Viral RNA-Dependent RNA Polymerases Using a Function-Site Interaction Fingerprint Method for RNA Virus Drug Discovery. J Proteome Res **2020,** *19* (11), 4698-4705.

[58] Zhao, Z.; Bourne, P. E., Revealing Acquired Resistance Mechanisms of Kinase-Targeted Drugs Using an on-the-Fly, Function-Site Interaction Fingerprint Approach. J Chem Theory Comput **2020,** *16* (5), 3152-3161.

[59] Liao, J. J., Molecular recognition of protein kinase binding pockets for design of potent and selective kinase inhibitors. J Med Chem **2007,** *50* (3), 409-424.

[60] Sordella, R.; Bell, D. W.; Haber, D. A.; Settleman, J., Gefitinib-sensitizing EGFR mutations in lung cancer activate anti-apoptotic pathways. Science **2004,** *305* (5687), 1163-1167.

[61] Gajiwala, K. S.; Feng, J.; Ferre, R.; Ryan, K.; Brodsky, O.; Weinrich, S.; Kath, J. C.; Stewart, A., Insights into the aberrant activity of mutant EGFR kinase domain and drug recognition. Structure **2013,** *21* (2), 209-219.

[62] Leproult, E.; Barluenga, S.; Moras, D.; Wurtz, J. M.; Winssinger, N., Cysteine mapping in conformationally distinct kinase nucleotide binding sites: application to the design of selective covalent inhibitors. J Med Chem **2011,** *54* (5), 1347-1355.

[63] Zhao, Z.; Liu, Q.; Bliven, S.; Xie, L.; Bourne, P. E., Determining Cysteines Available for Covalent Inhibition Across the Human Kinome. J Med Chem **2017,** *60* (7), 2879-2889.

[64] Lin, J. J.; Riely, G. J.; Shaw, A. T., Targeting ALK: Precision Medicine Takes on Drug Resistance. Cancer Discov **2017,** *7* (2), 137-155.

[65] Baldo, B. A.; Pham, N. H., Adverse reactions to targeted and non-targeted chemotherapeutic drugs with emphasis on hypersensitivity responses and the invasive metastatic switch. Cancer Metastasis Rev **2013,** *32* (3-4), 723-761.

[66] O'Brien, S. G.; Guilhot, F.; Larson, R. A.; Gathmann, I.; Baccarani, M.; Cervantes, F.; Cornelissen, J. J.; Fischer, T.; Hochhaus, A.; Hughes, T.; Lechner, K.; Nielsen, J. L.; Rousselot, P.; Reiffers, J.; Saglio, G.; Shepherd, J.; Simonsson, B.; Gratwohl, A.; Goldman, J. M.; Kantarjian, H.; Taylor, K.; Verhoef, G.; Bolton, A. E.; Capdeville, R.; Druker, B. J.; Investigators, I., Imatinib compared with interferon and low-dose cytarabine for newly diagnosed chronic-phase chronic myeloid leukemia. *N Engl J Med* **2003,** *348* (11), 994-1004.

[67] Dy, G. K.; Adjei, A. A., Understanding, recognizing, and managing toxicities of targeted anticancer therapies. CA Cancer J Clin **2013,** *63* (4), 249-279.

[68] Posy, S. L.; Hermsmeier, M. A.; Vaccaro, W.; Ott, K. H.; Todderud, G.; Lippy, J. S.; Trainor, G. L.; Loughney, D. A.; Johnson, S. R., Trends in kinase selectivity: insights for target class-focused library screening. J Med Chem **2011,** *54* (1), 54-66.

[69] Aldeghi, M.; Gapsys, V.; de Groot, B. L., Predicting Kinase Inhibitor Resistance: Physics-Based and Data-Driven Approaches. ACS Cent Sci **2019,** *5* (8), 1468-1474.

[70] Yun, C. H.; Mengwasser, K. E.; Toms, A. V.; Woo, M. S.; Greulich, H.; Wong, K. K.; Meyerson, M.; Eck, M. J., The T790M mutation in EGFR kinase causes drug resistance by increasing the affinity for ATP. Proc Natl Acad Sci U S A **2008,** *105* (6), 2070-2075.

[71] Katayama, R.; Shaw, A. T.; Khan, T. M.; Mino-Kenudson, M.; Solomon, B. J.; Halmos, B.; Jessop, N. A.; Wain, J. C.; Yeo, A. T.; Benes, C.; Drew, L.; Saeh, J. C.; Crosby, K.; Sequist, L. V.; Iafrate, A. J.; Engelman, J. A., Mechanisms of acquired crizotinib resistance in ALK-rearranged lung Cancers. *Sci Transl Med* **2012,** *4* (120), 120ra17.

[72] Weisberg, E.; Boulton, C.; Kelly, L. M.; Manley, P.; Fabbro, D.; Meyer, T.; Gilliland, D. G.; Griffin, J. D., Inhibition of mutant FLT3 receptors in leukemia cells by the small molecule tyrosine kinase inhibitor PKC412. Cancer Cell **2002,** *1* (5), 433-443.

[73] Wu, Y. L.; Zhang, L.; Kim, D. W.; Liu, X.; Lee, D. H.; Yang, J. C.; Ahn, M. J.; Vansteenkiste, J. F.; Su, W. C.; Felip, E.; Chia, V.; Glaser, S.; Pultar, P.; Zhao, S.; Peng, B.; Akimov, M.; Tan, D. S. W., Phase Ib/II Study of Capmatinib (INC280) Plus Gefitinib After Failure of

Epidermal Growth Factor Receptor (EGFR) Inhibitor Therapy in Patients With EGFR-Mutated, MET Factor-Dysregulated Non-Small-Cell Lung Cancer. J Clin Oncol **2018,** *36* (31), 3101-3109.

[74] Vamathevan, J.; Clark, D.; Czodrowski, P.; Dunham, I.; Ferran, E.; Lee, G.; Li, B.; Madabhushi, A.; Shah, P.; Spitzer, M.; Zhao, S., Applications of machine learning in drug discovery and development. Nat Rev Drug Discov **2019,** *18* (6), 463-477.

[75] Dunn, M. C.; Bourne, P. E., Building the biomedical data science workforce. PLoS Biol **2017,** *15* (7), e2003082.

[76] Coley, C. W.; Green, W. H.; Jensen, K. F., Machine Learning in Computer-Aided Synthesis Planning. Acc Chem Res **2018,** *51* (5), 1281-1289.

[77] Bagherian, M.; Sabeti, E.; Wang, K.; Sartor, M. A.; Nikolovska-Coleska, Z.; Najarian, K., Machine learning approaches and databases for prediction of drug-target interaction: a survey paper. Brief Bioinform **2021,** *22* (1), 247-269.

[78] Christmann-Franck, S.; van Westen, G. J.; Papadatos, G.; Beltran Escudie, F.; Roberts, A.; Overington, J. P.; Domine, D., Unprecedently Large-Scale Kinase Inhibitor Set Enabling the Accurate Prediction of Compound-Kinase Activities: A Way toward Selective Promiscuity by Design? J Chem Inf Model **2016,** *56* (9), 1654-1675.

[79] Sorgenfrei, F. A.; Fulle, S.; Merget, B., Kinome-Wide Profiling Prediction of Small Molecules. ChemMedChem **2018,** *13* (6), 495-499.

[80] Li, X.; Li, Z.; Wu, X.; Xiong, Z.; Yang, T.; Fu, Z.; Liu, X.; Tan, X.; Zhong, F.; Wan, X.; Wang, D.; Ding, X.; Yang, R.; Hou, H.; Li, C.; Liu, H.; Chen, K.; Jiang, H.; Zheng, M., Deep Learning Enhancing Kinome-Wide Polypharmacology Profiling: Model Construction and Experiment Validation. J Med Chem **2020,** *63* (16), 8723-8737.

[81] Miljkovic, F.; Bajorath, J., Data structures for computational compound promiscuity analysis and exemplary applications to inhibitors of the human kinome. J Comput Aided Mol Des **2020,** *34* (1), 1-10.

Chapter 4

Time Series Analysis on the Conformational Change of c-Src Tyrosine Kinase

Hyun Jung Yoon, Sungmin Lee, Suhyun Park and Sangwook Wu

Abstract

c-Src tyrosine kinase plays an important role in signal transduction pathways, where its activity is regulated by phosphorylation of the two tyrosine residues. We performed targeted molecular dynamics simulation to obtain trajectory of conformational change from inactive to active form. To investigate the conformational change of c-Src tyrosine kinase, we applied network analysis to time series of correlation among residues. The time series of correlation between residues during the conformational change generated by targeted molecular dynamic simulation. With centrality measures such as betweenness centrality, degree centrality, and closeness centrality, we observed a few important residues that significantly contribute to the conformational change of c-Src tyrosine kinase for the different time steps.

Keywords: c-Src tyrosine kinase, targeted molecular dynamics simulation, network analysis, time-series, clustering

1. Introduction

Tyrosine kinases play a critical role in various biological processes such as migration, angiogenesis, proliferation, differentiation, survival, and immune function [1–3]. c-Src (cellular Src), encoded by Src gene, is a non-receptor tyrosine kinase first isolated as the normal cellular homolog to the potent avian sarcoma viral transforming oncogene v-Src [4]. c-Src tyrosine kinase consists of the N-terminal unique region, the Src homology 3 (SH3), SH2, linker, kinase domain, and the regulatory C-terminal tail. Under normal circumstances, the SH3 domain of the c-Src tyrosine kinase binds to the proline-rich region in the linker domain. And the SH2 domain binds to Tyr527, which leads to a closed conformation [5, 6]. However, under certain conditions, the closed, inactive c-Src tyrosine kinase undergoes a transition to an open and active conformation. One of the important features of c-Src tyrosine kinase catalytic activation is to control its phosphorylation status. One of the major phosphorylation sites is Tyr527, which is located in the C-terminal tail. Dephosphorylation of pTyr527 (phosphorylated Tyr527) releases the closed conformation, which leads to the active state. Another major phosphorylation site is Tyr416, which is located in the activation loop of the tyrosine kinase domain [7, 8]. c-Src tyrosine kinase activity depends on the phosphorylation status of the two residues: Tyr527 and the Tyr416.

Using targeted molecular dynamics (TMD) simulation, we study the conformational change of c-Src tyrosine kinase by applying an external bias [9]. We generate sequential and continuous transition between two known conformations: the inactive and the active conformation for the case of Tyr527-pTyr416 (instead of pTyr527-Tyr416).

Network analysis has been successfully applied to biological problems [10, 11]. For instance, Goh et al. constructed a network of Mendelian gene-disease associations to identify unknown important genes causing disease [12]. In a biological network, a node corresponds to a gene and an edge is an interaction or correlation between genes. Centrality measures are very effective approaches to determine the ranking or importance of genes in the gene-disease network. Those centrality measures uncover important target genes relevant to disease. In this study, using network analysis, clustering method, and time-series analysis, we attempt to reveal the key residues, which influence the conformational transition of the c-Src tyrosine kinase between the inactive and active conformation.

2. Method

2.1 Targeted molecular dynamics (TMD) simulation

To perform the Targeted Molecular Dynamics simulation, an external potential, U_{TMD} [13], to be defined.

$$U_{TMD} = \frac{k}{2N}\left[RMSD(t) - RMSD^*(t)\right]^2 \tag{1}$$

In the above equation, RMSD(t) is defined as root-mean-square deviation (RMSD) of the simulated structure from the target structure at time t. RMSD*(t) is the RMSD value at time t assuming a linear decrease from the initial to the target structure. The inactive (PDB ID: 2SRC) and active form (PDB id: 1Y57) of c-Src tyrosine kinase are defined as initial and target conformation, respectively [14, 15]. Both the conformations were modified (to have the same number of atoms) for the TMD simulation. The spring constant '*k*' was set as 2500 kcal/mol $\cdot$Å^2 for 3,619 atoms (hydrogen atoms excluded). NAMD 2.9 [16] with the CHARMM 27 force field [17] was used to perform simulation and the protein parameters were incorporated with the CMAP corrections [18]. In TMD, the conformational change from inactive to the active state is guided by the external force within a reasonable time scale. In our calculation, we have used 10 ns time scale. To undergo the conformational change within 10 ns time scale and to avoid the bias effect, we employed the smallest spring constant 'k' (2500 kcal/mol $\cdot$Å^2). TIP3P water model [19] was used in the simulation. The particle mesh Ewald (PME) method was set as 12 Å direct space cut-off [20]. The damping coefficient was set as 5 ps^{-1} for the Langevin dynamics simulation. To maintain the constant pressure (1 atm), Nosé–Hoover method was used (1 atm) [21]. The NPT ensemble was carried out in 310K for the TMD simulation.

2.2 Network analysis

To analyze the correlation between residues in the trajectories of the TMD simulations, we have used the dynamical cross-correlation (DCCM) method [22–24].

$$C_{ij} = \frac{<(r_i(t) - <r_i(t)>)(r_j(t) - <r_j(t)>)>}{\sqrt{(<r_i^2(t)> - <r_i(t)>^2)(<r_j^2(t)> - <r_j(t)>^2)}} \tag{2}$$

Where, $r_i(t)$ and $r_j(t)$ = atomic positions of the ith and j^{th} C_α atoms at time t. The quantity "$r_i(t) - <r_i(t)>$" corresponds to the fluctuation of the "i^{th}" atom and "$r_j(t) - <r_j(t)>$" corresponds to the fluctuation of the "j^{th}" atom. For all the Cα atoms, a 450 × 450 (residues 84-533) correlation map was obtained during the 10 ns TMD simulation. In Eq. (2), the quantity C_{ij} in the DCCM is an adjacency matrix. The weight w_{ij}, of the edge between the nodes, 'i and j', defined as [25, 26]

$$w_{ij} = -log\,|C_{ij}| \tag{3}$$

DCCM can be used to measure the weight, which is the probability of information transfer across the edge. In the constructed network, every node is a Cα atom and each edge is an information transfer probability, in the cross-correlation. To identify and quantify the nodes that occupy critical positions in a network, a few centrality measures have been proposed, including the degree, betweenness, and closeness centralities [27–29].

The degree centrality measures the number of edges incident on a node in a network, thus expressing the "popularity" of the node.

$$C_D(v_i) = d_i = \sum_j A_{ij} \tag{4}$$

where A_{ij} is the adjacency matrix: if w_{ij} = 0 then A_{ij} = 0, otherwise A_{ij} = 1. The closeness centrality is defined as the average length of the shortest paths between a node and all the other nodes in a network. It can be used to measure information spread from a given node to the other nodes. The closeness centrality is defined as

$$C_C(v_i) = \frac{n-1}{\sum_{j \neq i} g(v_i, v_j)} \tag{5}$$

where $g(v_i, v_j)$ is the shortest path with a weight between two nodes 'i' and 'j'. The betweenness centrality is to measure the number of information pathways that flow through a node in a network. The betweenness of node 'i' is the fraction of the shortest paths between pairs of nodes that pass through node 'i'. The betweenness centrality is defined as

$$b_i = \frac{\sum_{s<t} g_i^{st} / n_{st}}{\frac{1}{2} n(n-1)} \tag{6}$$

where g_i^{st} is the number of shortest paths from 's' to 't' with a weight that passes through node 'i'. n_{st} is the total number of shortest paths from to 's' to 't'. We obtained DCCM and three centralities using Bio3d [30–32]

2.3 Clustering

Clustering is an effective approach to discover interesting patterns of time series data. It is widely used in diverse fields of research from biology to economy: functional clustering of time-series gene expression data [33], identification of functionally related genes [34–36], detecting brain activity [37, 38], identifying pathological cases from mass spectrometry (MS) clinical samples [39], discovering energy consumption pattern [40, 41], and pattern finding in stock time series [42, 43].

Using the targeted molecular simulation (TMD), we generated a dynamical correlation matrix between two residues, C_{ij}, for each time step during the conformational change from the inactive to active state. Then, the time-series of C_{ij} are grouped into a set of time series in such a way that their temporal profiles in the same group (cluster) are more similar to each other than those in other groups (clusters). We applied a hierarchical clustering algorithm and repeated clustering runs with a different number of clusters from 4 to 10 until getting clear clustering. The function 'tsclust [44]' of 'DTWclust [45]' in the R statistical package is used for clustering of time series data.

3. Results and discussion

3.1 Conformational change of c-Src tyrosine kinase

The electrostatic interaction between the Tyr527 and the positively charged Arg175/Lys203 becomes weaker in the inactive conformation at the early stage of the transition from the inactive to the active conformation by TMD simulation. The C-terminal tail, including Tyr527, is completely detached from the SH2 domain (the period of 0-3 ns) in the TMD simulation. The detachment of Tyr527 from the SH2 domain triggers the conformational change. The detached Tyr527 moves toward the kinase domain (4-6 ns period: **Figure 1b** and **c**). At this stage, the most prominent conformational change occurs in the kinase domain. The secondary structures,

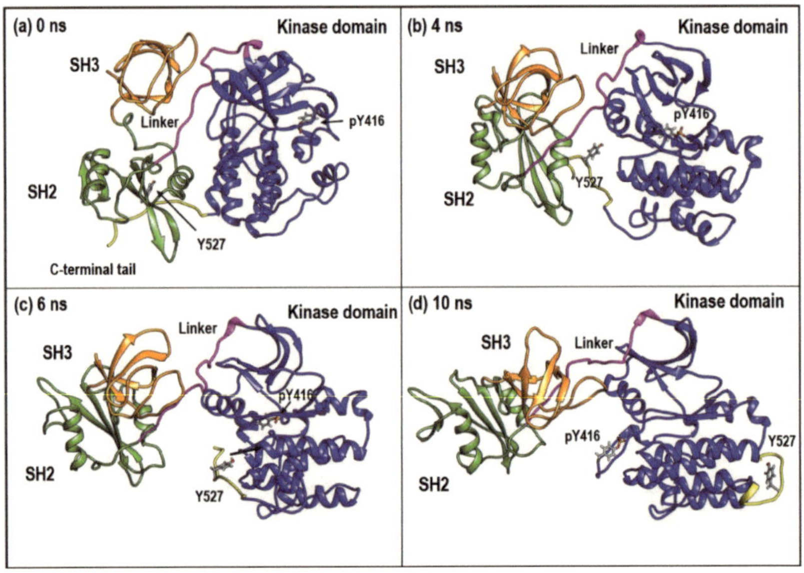

Figure 1.
Four snapshots of TMD simulation of c-Src tyrosine kinase between 0 and 10 ns. (a) 0 ns: inactive conformation (b) 4 ns: Detachment of Tyr527 in the C-terminal tail from the SH2 domain (c) 6 ns: Large-scale conformational change of c-Src tyrosine kinase (d) 10 ns: active conformation. Color code: SH3 (resid 84-142, Orange), SH2 (resid 143-245, Green), linker (resid 246-266, Magenta), and tyrosine kinase domains (resid 267-520, Blue), the regulatory C-terminal tail (resid 521-533, Yellow). The two residues, pTyr416 and Tyr527, are represented as licorice [9].

including the αC-helix in the kinase domain, rotate significantly. During this time, Tyr416 remains buried beneath the activation loop. At the final stage of transition, Tyr527 has reached the far side of the kinase domain relative to the SH2 domain. The activation loop has also moved from its original position. pTyr416 is now exposed to the surface.

The activation processes from the inactive state (0 ns: **Figure 1a**) to the active state (10 ns: **Figure 1d**) in the TMD simulation are shown in **Figure 1**. The conformational transition of c-Src tyrosine kinase from the inactive to the active state generated by TMD simulation is shown in the supplementary video material [9].

3.2 Centrality measures

The degree, closeness, and betweenness centralities are measured for the conformational change that occurred during the 10 ns TMD simulation (**Figure 2**). The residues with high values of the degree, closeness, and betweenness centralities are not located in the activation loop, linker, αC-helix. The residues with high centrality measures are mainly confined to the helix region adjacent to the αC-helix. The residues with the top 5 values of each centrality measure are listed in **Table 1**.

3.3 Clustering

We investigate correlation patterns between specific residues (Trp260, Tyr416, Tyr527, Lys321) and all the other residues using the clustering method. The clustering of residues provides us with information on not only the pattern of the time series but also the correlation values, C_{ij}, between residues at each time step.

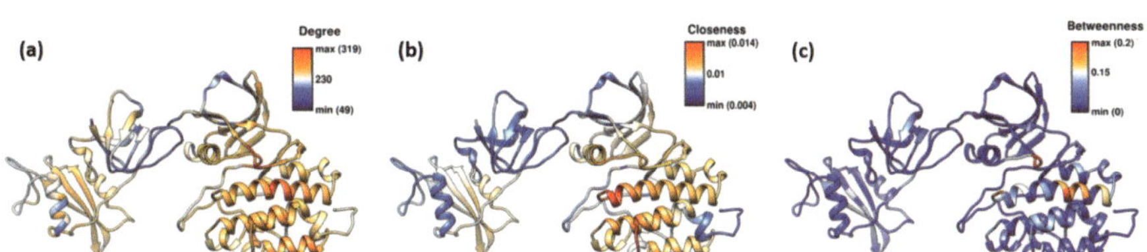

Figure 2.
Centrality measures during the 10 ns TMD simulation. (a) Degree centrality (b) Closeness centrality (c) Betweenness centrality. We mapped centrality measures onto the active conformation of c-Src tyrosine kinase [9].

	Betweenness	Closeness	Degree
1	Glu320	Val377	Val323
2	Lys321	Arg379	Val402
3	Ala368	Glu378	Lys321
4	Leu322	Met380	Ile370
5	Met380	Thr508	Thr301

Table 1.
Top 5 residues of each centrality measure [9].

3.3.1 Trp260

Trp260 has an important role in the conformational change of c-Src tyrosine kinase [46]. **Figure 3** shows a time series of correlation, C_{ij} (t), for Trp260. It shows distinctive patterns among clustering groups. Residues in both group 6 (**Figure 3a**) and group 11 (**Figure 3b**) are positively correlated to Trp260 for the entire time window (0-10 ns). The residues in clustering group 9 (**Figure 3c**), however, are negatively correlated to Trp260. **Figure 1a** shows no correlation in early time (0-4 ns). The correlation increases positively (4-7 ns), and reaches the highest correlation value (~7 ns). Eventually, the correlation decreases (8-10 ns). The location of residues in clustering group 6 (orchid), clustering group 9 (cyan), and clustering group 11 (pink) are shown (**Figure 3d**). The positively correlated (blue) and negatively correlated residues (red) are shown (**Figure 3e**). The positively correlated residues are mainly located near residue Trp260 in the inactive form of c-Src tyrosine kinase. The negatively correlated residues are spread around a relatively far from Trp260 in the inactive form. The time series analysis based on the clustering method and network analysis indicates that Trp260 is rapidly changing its position after the second half of the conformational transition.

3.3.2 pTyr416

Figure 4 shows the time series of correlation, C_{ij} (t), for pTyr416. The residues in the clustering group 12 are positively correlated to Tyr416 for the entire time

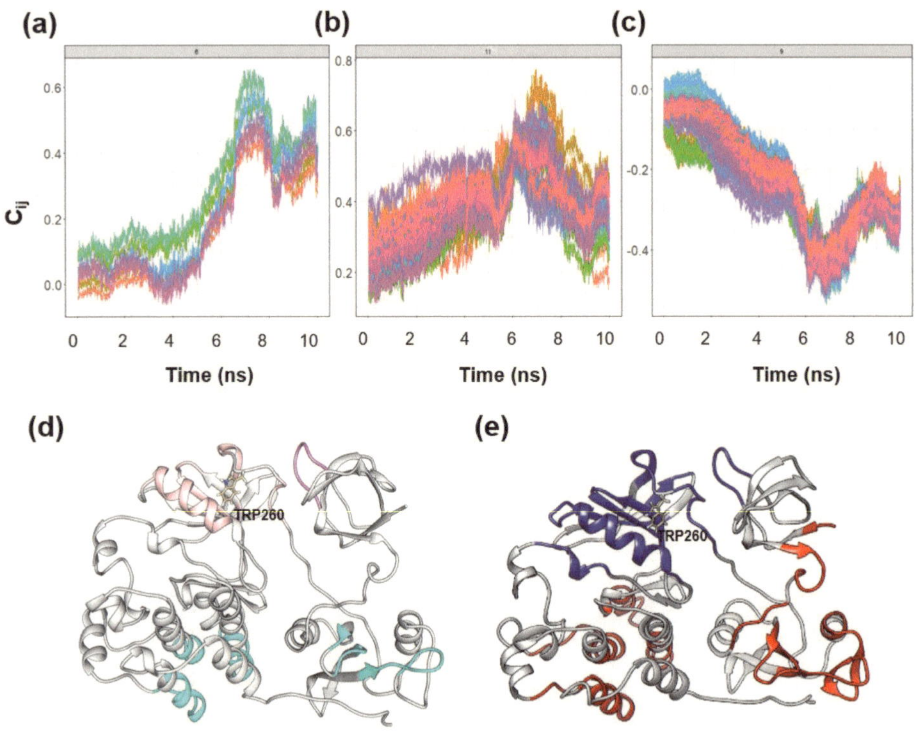

Figure 3.
Some distinctive clusters on the time series of correlation between Trp260 and other residues. (a) Clustering group 6 (b) Clustering group 11 (c) Clustering group 9 (d) Each cluster is mapped on the inactive conformation. Color code: orchid, pink and cyan for clustering 6, 11, and 9 respectively. (e) The positive correlation clusters (blue) and negative correlation clusters (red) on the inactive conformation.

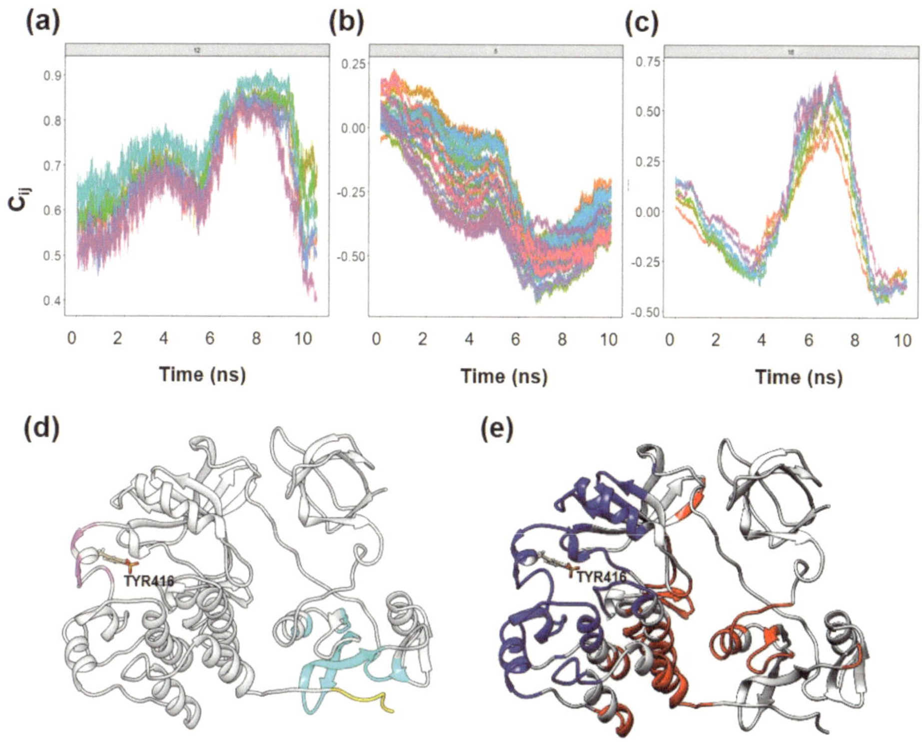

Figure 4.
Some distinctive clusters on the time series of correlation between pTyr416 and other residues. (a) Clustering group 12 (b) Clustering group 5 (c) Clustering group 16 (d) Each cluster is mapped on the inactive conformation. Color code: orchid, cyan, and yellow for clustering 12, 5, and 16 respectively. (e) The positive correlation clusters (blue) and negative correlation clusters (red) on the inactive conformation.

window (0-10 ns) (**Figure 4a**). The residues in the clustering group 5, however, are negatively correlated to pTyr416 (**Figure 4b**). Interestingly, the residues in the clustering group 16 show correlation change in the two different time regimes (**Figure 4c**). As shown in **Figure 4a**, C_{ij} (t) has a large value (> 0.5) even in early time and increases to 0.9. During the 7-8 ns period, C_{ij} (t) reaches a plateau with the highest correlation value. After 8 ns, C_{ij} (t) returns to 0.5. The residues in the clustering group 12, shown in orchid in **Figure 4d**, are mainly located close to pTyr416. The positive correlation between the clustering group 12 and pTyr416 is due to "physical distance".

Most of the residues in the clustering group 5 are negatively correlated to pTyr416 during the conformational transition (**Figure 4b**). C_{ij} (t) decreases to a minimum value of -0.7 around 7 ns and returns to -0.3. The residues in group 5, shown as cyan in **Figure 4d**, are located far away from pTyr416. The negative value of C_{ij} (t) indicates that the movement of pTyr416 and the residues in the clustering group 5 are in a reverse direction.

The residues in the clustering group 16 show the correlation pattern change to pTyr416 during the conformational transition. During 0-4 ns period, residues in group 16 (shown as yellow in **Figure 4d**) shows negatively correlated to pTyr416 with a minimum value of -0.3 in C_{ij} (t). And after 4 ns, the correlation pattern shows positively correlated to pTyr416. C_{ij} (t) reaches 0.7 around 7 ns in the conformational transition process.

The positively correlated (blue) and negatively correlated residues (red) to pTyr416 are mapped into the inactive conformation (**Figure 4e**).

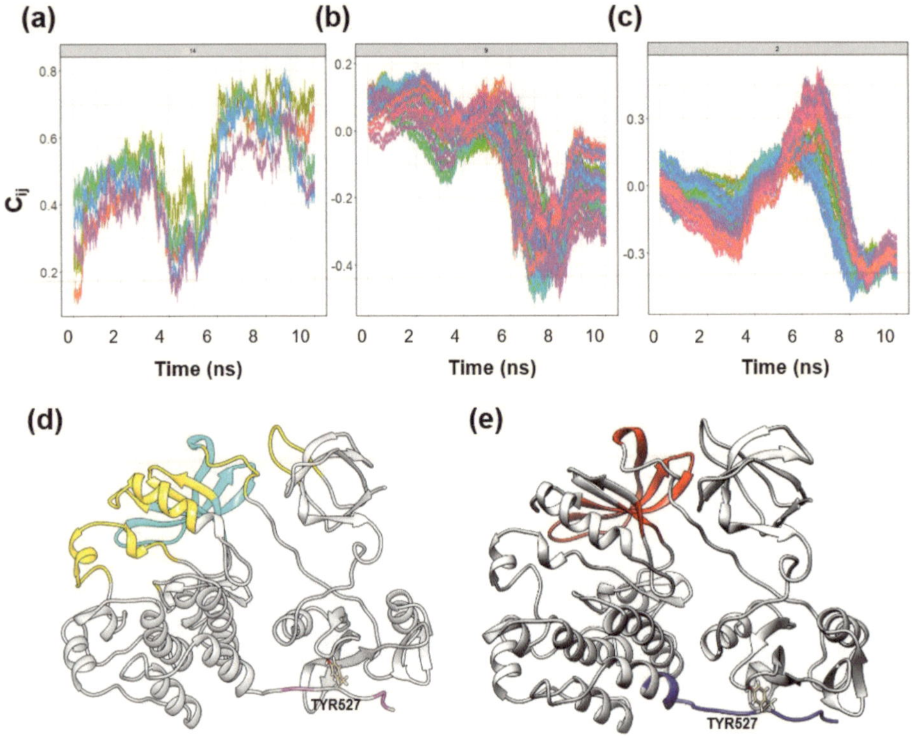

Figure 5.
Some distinctive clusters on the time series of correlation between pTyr416 and other residues.
(a) Clustering group 14 (b) Clustering group 9 (c) Clustering group 2 (d) Each cluster is mapped on the inactive conformation. Color code: orchid, cyan, and yellow for clustering 14, 9, and 2 respectively. (e) The positive correlation clusters (blue) and negative correlation clusters (red) on the inactive conformation.

3.3.3 Tyr527

Figure 5 shows the time series of correlation, C_{ij} (t), for Tyr527. The residues in the clustering group 14 are positively correlated to Tyr527 for the entire time window (0-10 ns) (**Figure 5a**). The residues in the clustering group 9, however, are negatively correlated to Tyr527 during the most time of conformational transition (**Figure 4b**). As with the case of pTyr416, the residues in the clustering group 2 show correlation pattern change in the two different time regimes (**Figure 5c**). As shown in **Figure 5a**, C_{ij} (t) increases to 0.6 during 0-4 ns period. After an abrupt decrease, C_{ij} (t) increases again to reach a plateau with the value of 0.6 during 6-10 ns. The residues in the clustering group 14 (shown as orchid in **Figure 5d**) are located close to Tyr527. Similarly, the positive correlation between the clustering group 14 and Tyr527 is due to a strong coupled through "physical distance".

Most of the residues in the clustering group 9 are negatively correlated to Tyr527 during the conformational transition (**Figure 5b**). The residues in the clustering group 9 (shown as cyan in **Figure 5d**) are located away from Tyr527 in the inactive conformation.

The residues in the clustering group 2 show the correlation pattern change to Tyr527 during the conformational transition, which is observed in the case of pTyr416. During 0-4 ns period, the residues in the clustering group 2 (shown as yellow in **Figure 5d**) shows negatively correlated to Tyr527 with a minimum value of -0.3 in C_{ij} (t). And after 4 ns, the correlation pattern shows positively correlated to Tyr527. In the last, C_{ij} (t) reaches 0.45 around 7 ns in the conformational transition process.

The positively correlated (blue) and negatively correlated residues (red) to pTyr416 are mapped into the inactive conformation (**Figure 5e**).

3.3.4 Lys321

According to network analysis, Lys321 has high centralities both in betweenness and degree centralities (**Table 1**). Within the framework of network theory, it implies that Lys321 would play an essential role in the conformational change of c-Src tyrosine kinase. The residues in the clustering group 13 are positively correlated to Lys321 for the entire time window (0-10 ns) (**Figure 6a**). The residues in the clustering group 1 are negatively correlated to Lys321 (**Figure 6b**). As with the cases of pTyr416 and Tyr527, the residues in the clustering group 16 show correlation pattern change in the two different time regimes (**Figure 6c**).

As shown in **Figure 6a**, C_{ij} (t) values fluctuate around 0.5 during the 0-5 ns period. After that, it increases to 0.7 around 7 ns. Finally, it decreases to around 0.55. The residues in the clustering group 13 (shown as an orchid in **Figure 6d**) are located close to Lys 321. Similarly, the positive correlation between the clustering group 14 and Lys321 is due to a strong coupled through "physical distance".

Most of the residues in the clustering group 1 are negatively correlated to Lys321 during the conformational transition (**Figure 6b**). The residues in the clustering group 1 (shown as cyan in **Figure 5d**) are located away from Lys321 in the inactive conformation. **Figure 6b** shows that C_{ij} decreases to -0.5 until 6 ns and increases and

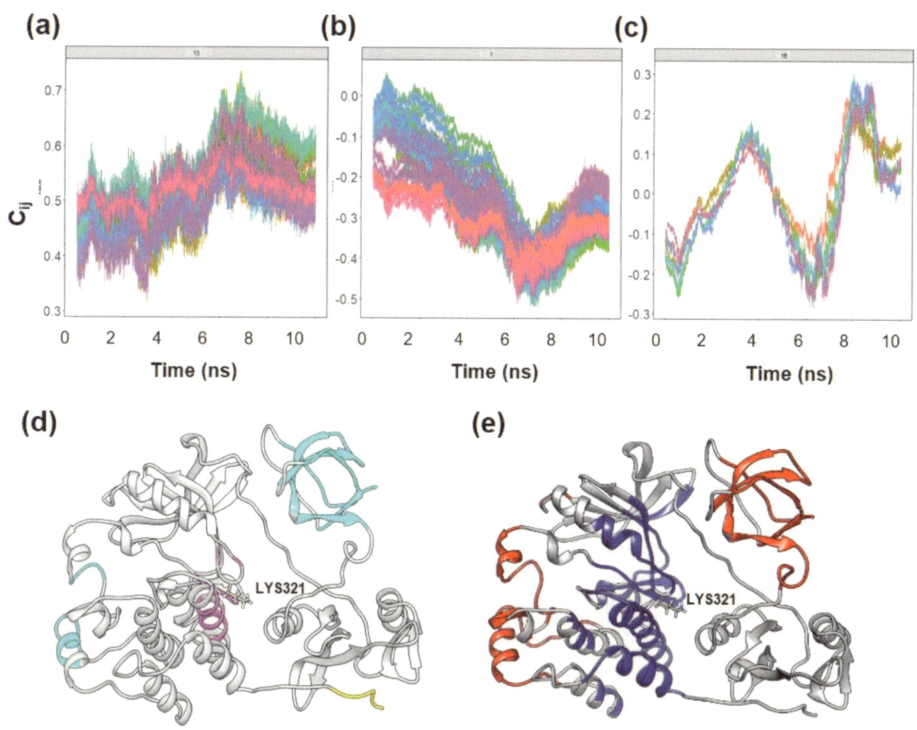

Figure 6.
Some distinctive clusters on the time series of correlation between Lys321and other residues. (a) Clustering group 13 (b) Clustering group 1 (c) Clustering group 16 (d) Each cluster is mapped on the inactive conformation. Color code: orchid, cyan, and yellow for clustering 13, 1, and 16 respectively. (e) The positive correlation clusters (blue) and negative correlation clusters (red) on the inactive conformation.

TRP260	Positive correlation	Cluster 6	93, 94, 95, 96, 97, 98, 99
	Positive correlation	Cluster 11	253, 254, 255, 256, 257, 263, 264, 265, 266, 267, 303, 304, 305, 306, 307, 308, 309, 310, 311, 312, 313, 314, 315, 325, 326, 330, 331, 332, 333, 334, 335, 336, 337
	Negative correlation	Cluster 9	176, 177, 180, 181, 182, 183, 184, 185, 203, 204, 205, 206, 207, 208, 209, 210, 211, 212, 213, 355, 356, 357, 358, 359, 360, 361, 362, 363, 364, 365, 366, 367, 452, 453, 454, 455, 456, 457, 458, 483, 484, 485, 486, 487, 488, 489, 490, 491, 492, 493, 494, 495
TYR416	Positive correlation	Cluster 12	413, 414, 418, 419, 420, 424
	Negative correlation	Cluster 5	162, 163, 169, 170, 171, 172, 173, 174, 184, 185, 186, 187, 188, 189, 190, 191, 192, 193, 194, 195, 196, 197, 198, 199, 200, 201, 202, 203, 204, 205, 214, 215, 236, 237, 238, 239
	Switch	Cluster 16	527, 528, 529, 530, 531, 532, 533
TYR527	Positive correlation	Cluster 14	524, 525, 530, 531, 532
	Negative correlation	Cluster 9	263, 264, 265, 266, 267, 268, 269, 270, 271, 272, 273, 274, 275, 276, 277, 278, 279, 280, 281, 282, 283, 284, 285, 286, 287, 288, 289, 290, 291, 292, 293, 294, 295, 296, 325, 326, 337, 338, 339, 340
	Switch	Cluster 2	93, 94, 95, 96, 97, 98, 99, 100, 101, 255, 256, 257, 258, 259, 260, 261, 262, 297, 298, 299, 300, 301, 302, 303, 304, 305, 306, 307, 308, 309, 310, 311, 312, 313, 327, 328, 329, 330, 331, 332, 333, 334, 335, 336, 386, 405, 406, 407, 408, 409, 410, 411, 412, 413, 414, 415, 416, 417, 418, 419, 420, 421, 422, 423, 424
LYS321	Positive correlation	Cluster 13	319, 323, 368, 369, 370, 371, 372, 374, 375, 376, 399, 400, 402
	Negative correlation	Cluster 1	84, 85, 86, 87, 88, 89, 99, 100, 101, 102, 103, 104, 105, 106, 107, 108, 109, 110, 111, 112, 113, 118, 119, 120, 121, 122, 123, 124, 125, 126, 127, 128, 129, 130, 131, 132, 133, 134, 136, 137, 138, 139, 140, 420, 421, 422, 423, 424, 466, 467, 468, 469, 470, 471, 472, 473, 474
	Switch	Cluster 16	528, 529, 530, 531, 532, 533

Table 2.
*The residues in the clustering group (**Figures 3d, 4d, 5d, and 6d**).*

reaches -0.3 at the end of the conformational transition. The residues in the clustering group 1, shown in purple in **Figure 6d**, are located quite away from Lys321.

The residues in the clustering group 16 show the correlation pattern change to Lys321 during the conformational transition, which is observed in the cases of pTyr416 and Tyr527. During 0-2 ns period, the residues in the clustering group 16 (shown as yellow in **Figure 6d**) shows negatively correlated to Lys321 with the minimum value of -0.25 in C_{ij} (t). And for 2-4 ns, the correlation pattern shows positively correlated to Lys321. After 4 ns, it sharply decreases to the minimum value of -0.25. Subsequently, it reaches the maximum positive value of 0.3 in C_{ij} (t). Eventually, it decreases to zero. The C_{ij} (t) for Lys321 shows more correlation pattern changes compared to the cases of pTyr416 and Tyr527.

The positively correlated (blue) and negatively correlated residues (red) to Lys321 are mapped into the inactive conformation (**Figure 6e**).

The residues in the clustering group (**Figures 3d, 4d, 5d**, and **6d**) are listed in **Table 2** positively and negatively correlated residues in the clustering group (**Figures 3e, 4e, 5e**, and **6e**) are listed in **Table 3**.

TRP260	Negative correlation	Cluster 1	84, 85, 86, 138, 139, 140, 141, 142, 143, 144, 145, 146, 149, 150, 151, 152, 153, 154, 174, 175, 178, 179, 186, 202, 214, 215, 216, 217, 218, 219, 220, 221, 222, 223, 224, 225, 226, 227, 346, 347, 348, 349, 350, 351, 352, 353, 354, 389, 448, 449, 450, 451, 459, 460, 461, 462, 463, 464, 465, 479, 480, 481, 482, 496, 497, 498, 499
		Cluster 9	176, 177, 180, 181, 182, 183, 184, 185, 203, 204, 205, 206, 207, 208, 209, 210, 211, 212, 213, 355, 356, 357, 358, 359, 360, 361, 362, 363, 364, 365, 366, 367, 452, 453, 454, 455, 456, 457, 458, 483, 484, 485, 486, 487, 488, 489, 490, 491, 492, 493, 494, 495
	Positive correlation	Cluster 6	93, 94, 95, 96, 97, 98, 99
		Cluster 10	:251, 252, 268, 284, 285, 286, 287, 288, 292, 293, 294, 295, 296, 297, 298, 299, 300, 301, 302, 316, 317, 318, 324, 338, 339, 406, 407, 408, 409, 410, 411, 412
		Cluster 11	253, 254, 255, 256, 257, 263, 264, 265, 266, 267, 303, 304, 305, 306, 307, 308, 309, 310, 311, 312, 313, 314, 315, 325, 326, 330, 331, 332, 333, 334, 335, 336, 337
		Cluster 12	258, 262, 327, 328, 329
		Cluster 13	259, 261
TYR416	Negative correlation	Cluster 4	149, 150, 151, 152, 153, 154, 155, 156, 157, 158, 159, 160, 161, 175, 176, 177, 178, 179, 180, 181, 182, 183, 208, 209, 210, 289, 290, 291, 320, 321, 339, 340, 341, 342, 343, 344, 346, 349, 350, 351, 352, 353, 367, 368, 369, 370, 372, 393, 394, 401, 452, 455, 456, 457, 458, 485, 486, 487, 488, 489, 490, 491, 492, 513, 514, 515, 516, 517, 518, 519, 520, 521, 522, 523
		Cluster 10	354, 355, 356, 357, 358, 359, 360, 361, 362, 363, 364, 365, 366, 395, 396, 397, 398, 399, 400
	Positive correlation	Cluster 6	261, 277, 278, 279, 296, 297, 298, 314, 328, 329, 330, 331, 332, 333, 334, 335, 336, 388, 404, 463, 466, 467
		Cluster 7	299, 300, 301, 302, 303, 304, 305, 306, 307, 308, 309, 310, 385, 386, 406, 407, 427, 428, 429, 430, 431, 432, 438, 439, 440, 443, 468, 469, 470, 471, 472, 473
		Cluster 8	311, 312, 313, 377, 378, 380, 381, 382, 383, 384, 387, 405, 441, 442, 444, 445, 446, 447, 474, 475, 476, 477, 478, 479, 499, 500, 501, 502, 503, 504, 505, 506
		Cluster 11	408, 409, 410, 411, 412, 421, 422, 423, 425, 426, 433, 434, 435, 436, 437
		Cluster 12	413, 414, 418, 419, 420, 424
		Cluster 13	415, 417
TYR527	Negative correlation	Cluster 9	263, 264, 265, 266, 267, 268, 269, 270, 271, 272, 273, 274, 275, 276, 277, 278, 279, 280, 281, 282, 283, 284, 285, 286, 287, 288, 289, 290, 291, 292, 293, 294, 295, 296, 325, 326, 337, 338, 339, 340
	Positive correlation	Cluster 13	516, 517, 518, 519, 520, 521, 522, 523, 533
		Cluster 14	524, 525, 530, 531, 532
		Cluster 15	526, 528, 529
LYS321	Negative correlation	Cluster 1	84, 85, 86, 87, 88, 89, 99, 100, 101, 102, 103, 104, 105, 106, 107, 108, 109, 110, 111, 112, 113, 118, 119, 120, 121, 122, 123, 124, 125, 126, 127, 128, 129, 130, 131, 132, 133, 134, 136, 137, 138, 139, 140, 420, 421, 422, 423, 424, 466, 467, 468, 469, 470, 471, 472, 473, 474

	Cluster 3	141, 142, 143, 144, 145, 146, 147, 298, 299, 300, 301, 413, 414, 415, 416, 417, 418, 419, 425, 426, 427, 428, 429, 431, 434, 435, 436, 460, 461, 462, 463, 464, 465, 475, 476, 477, 478, 479, 480, 481, 482
Positive correlation	Cluster 9	290, 291, 292, 293, 311, 312, 313, 327, 337, 345, 349, 358, 359, 360, 383, 384, 387, 389, 391, 404, 405, 441, 444, 445, 448, 490, 491, 494, 507
	Cluster 10	314, 315, 325, 326, 338, 340, 343, 344, 346, 381, 382
	Cluster 11	316, 339, 341, 342, 361, 362, 363, 380, 396, 397, 508, 515, 516, 517, 518, 519, 520, 521, 522
	Cluster 12	317, 318, 324, 364, 365, 366, 367, 377, 378, 379, 392, 393, 394, 395, 398, 403, 509, 510, 511, 512, 513, 514
	Cluster 13	319, 323, 368, 369, 370, 371, 372, 374, 375, 376, 399, 400, 402
	Cluster 14	320, 322, 373, 401

Table 3.
*Positively/negatively correlated residues in the clustering group (**Figures 3e, 4e, 5e, 6e**).*

4. Conclusions

In this study, we investigated the conformational transition of c-Src tyrosine kinase from the inactive to the active state using TMD simulation and network theory. Tyr416 and Tyr527 are known to be significant residues in the conformational transition by controlling the phosphorylation status. They play as a *switch* for the conversion of the inactive/active conformation. The time-dependent correlation matrices, C_{ij} (t), between all the residues and pTyr416 and Tyr527 show very similar patterns (positively correlated, negatively correlated, negatively/positively correlated) during the conformational transition process. The time-series analysis supports that pTrp416 and Tyr527 act as a *switch* in a very concerted manner for completion of conformational transition of c-Src tyrosine kinase. Based on the analysis of the three centrality measures (betweenness, closeness, and degree), we observed that Lys321 plays an essential role in the conformational transition of c-Src tyrosine kinase. The time-series analysis shows that C_{ij} (t), between all the residues and Lys321 show positively correlated, negatively correlated, and pattern change from negatively to positively correlated one during the conformational transition process. Combining the network analysis with time-series analysis, Lys321 may be another candidate for a *switch* for the conformational transition of c-Src tyrosine kinase.

Acknowledgements

This work was supported by the National Research Foundation of Korea(NRF) grant funded by the Korea government(MSIT) (NRF-2018R1D1A1B07048762).

Conflict of interest

The authors declare no conflict of interest.

Author details

Hyun Jung Yoon[1,2†], Sungmin Lee[1†], Suhyun Park[2] and Sangwook Wu[1,2*]

1 R&D Center of PharmCADD, Busan, Republic of Korea

2 Department of Physics, Pukyong National University, Busan, Republic of Korea

*Address all correspondence to: sangwoow@pknu.ac.kr; s.wu@pharmcadd.com

† These authors contributed equally.

References

[1] Frame MC. Newest findings on the oldest oncogene; how activated src does it. Journal of cell science. 2004;117(7): 989–998.

[2] Summy JM, Gallick GE. Treatment for advanced tumors: SRC reclaims center stage. Clinical Cancer Research. 2006;12(5):1398–1401.

[3] Yeatman TJ. A renaissance for SRC. Nature Reviews Cancer. 2004;4(6):470–480.

[4] Brown MT, Cooper JA. Regulation, substrates and functions of src. Biochimica et Biophysica Acta (BBA)-Reviews on Cancer. 1996;1287(2):121–149.

[5] Roskoski R. Src protein-tyrosine kinase structure, mechanism, and small molecule inhibitors. Pharmacological research. 2015;94:9–25.

[6] BOGGON TJ, ECK MJ. Structure and regulation of Src family kinases. Oncogene. 2004;23(48):7918–7927.

[7] Sun G, Sharma AK, Budde RJ. Autophosphorylation of Src and Yes blocks their inactivation by Csk phosphorylation. Oncogene. 1998;17 (12):1587–1595.

[8] Meng Y, Roux B. Locking the active conformation of c-Src kinase through the phosphorylation of the activation loop. Journal of molecular biology. 2014; 426(2):423–435.

[9] Yoon HJ, Lee S, Park SJ, Wu S. Network approach of the conformational change of c-Src, a tyrosine kinase, by molecular dynamics simulation. Scientific Reports. 2018;8 (1):5673.

[10] Ma'ayan A. Introduction to network analysis in systems biology. Science signaling. 2011;4(190):tr5–tr5.

[11] Almaas E. Biological impacts and context of network theory. Journal of Experimental Biology. 2007;210(9): 1548–1558.

[12] Goh KI, Cusick ME, Valle D, Childs B, Vidal M, Barabási AL. The human disease network. Proceedings of the National Academy of Sciences. 2007;104(21):8685–8690.

[13] Schlitter J, Engels M, Krüger P, Jacoby E, Wollmer A. Targeted molecular dynamics simulation of conformational change-application to the T↔R transition in insulin. Molecular Simulation. 1993;10(2-6):291–308.

[14] Xu W, Doshi A, Lei M, Eck MJ, Harrison SC. Crystal structures of c-Src reveal features of its autoinhibitory mechanism. Molecular cell.1999;3(5): 629–638.

[15] Cowan-Jacob SW, Fendrich G, Manley PW, Jahnke W, Fabbro D, Liebe-tanz J, et al. The crystal structure of a c-Src complex in an active conformation suggests possible steps in c-Src activation. Structure. 2005;13(6): 861–871.

[16] Phillips JC, Braun R, Wang W, Gumbart J, Tajkhorshid E, Villa E, et al. Scalable molecular dynamics with NAMD. Journal of computational chemistry. 2005;26(16):1781–1802.

[17] MacKerell AD, Banavali N, Foloppe N. Development and current status of the CHARMM force field for nucleic acids. Biopolymers. 2000;56(4): 257–265.

[18] MacKerell AD, Feig M, Brooks CL. Extending the treatment of back-bone energetics in protein force fields: Limitations of gas-phase quantum mechanics in reproducing protein conformational distributions in molecular dynamics simulations.

Journal of computational chemistry.2004;25(11):1400–1415.

[19] Jorgensen WL, Chandrasekhar J, Madura JD, Impey RW, Klein ML. Comparison of simple potential functions for simulating liquid water. The Journal of chemical physics. 1983;79 (2):926–935.

[20] Darden T, York D, Pedersen L. Particle mesh Ewald: An N·log (N) method for Ewald sums in large systems. The Journal of chemical physics. 1993;98(12):10089–10092.

[21] Feller SE, Zhang Y, Pastor RW, Brooks BR. Constant pressure molecular dynamics simulation: the Langevin piston method. The Journal of chemical physics. 1995;103(11): 4613–4621.

[22] Hünenberger P, Mark A, Van Gunsteren W. Fluctuation and cross-correlation analysis of protein motions observed in nanosecond molecular dynamics simulations. Journal of molecular biology. 1995;252(4):492–503.

[23] Karplus M, Ichiye T. Comment on a “fluctuation and cross correlation analysis of protein motions observed in nanosecond molecular dynamics simulations”. Elsevier; 1996.

[24] Kasahara K, Fukuda I, Nakamura H. A novel approach of dynamic cross correlation analysis on molecular dynamics simulations and its application to Ets1 dimer–DNA complex. PloS one. 2014;9(11):e112419.

[25] Sethi A, Eargle J, Black AA, Luthey-Schulten Z. Dynamical networks in tRNA: protein complexes. Proceedings of the National Academy of Sciences. 2009;106(16):6620–6625.

[26] VanWart AT, Eargle J, Luthey-Schulten Z, Amaro RE. Exploring residue component contributions to dynamical network models of allostery. Journal of chemical theory and computation. 2012;8(8):2949–2961.

[27] Freeman LC. Centrality in social networks conceptual clarification. Social networks. 1978;1(3):215–239.

[28] Mason O, Verwoerd M. Graph theory and networks in biology. IET systems biology. 2007;1(2):89–119.

[29] Newman ME. A measure of betweenness centrality based on random walks. Social networks. 2005;27 (1):39–54.

[30] Grant BJ, Rodrigues AP, ElSawy KM, McCammon JA, Caves LS. Bio3d: an R package for the comparative analysis of protein structures. Bioinformatics. 2006;22(21): 2695–2696.

[31] Skjærven L, Yao XQ, Scarabelli G, Grant BJ. Integrating protein structural dynamics and evolutionary analysis with Bio3D. BMC bioinformatics. 2014; 15(1):1–11.

[32] Skjærven L, Jariwala S, Yao XQ, Grant BJ. Online interactive analysis of protein structure ensembles with Bio3D-web. Bioinformatics. 2016;32 (22):3510–3512.

[33] Fujita A, Severino P, Kojima K, Sato JR, Patriota AG, Miyano S. Functional clustering of time series gene expression data by Granger causality. BMC systems biology. 2012;6(1):137.

[34] Möller-Levet CS, Klawonn F, Cho KH, Wolkenhauer O. Fuzzy clustering of short time-series and unevenly distributed sampling points. In: International Symposium on Intelligent Data Analysis. Springer; 2003. p. 330–340.

[35] Ernst J, Nau GJ, Bar-Joseph Z. Clustering short time series gene expression data. Bioinformatics. 2005;21 (suppl1):i159–i168.

[36] Pyatnitskiy M, Mazo I, Shkrob M, Schwartz E, Kotelnikova E. Clustering gene expression regulators: new approach to disease subtyping. PLoS One. 2014;9(1):e84955.

[37] Wang X, Nagarajan MB, Abidin AZ, DSouza A, Hobbs SK, Wismüller A. Investigating the use of mutual information and non-metric clustering for functional connectivity analysis on resting-state functional MRI. In: Medical Imaging 2015: Biomedical Applications in Molecular, Structural, and Functional Imaging. vol. 9417. International Society for Optics and Photonics; 2015. p. 94171N.

[38] Van Den Heuvel M, Mandl R, Pol HH. Normalized cut group clustering of resting-state FMRI data. PloS one. 2008;3(4):e2001.

[39] Gullo F, Ponti G, Tagarelli A, Tradigo G, Veltri P. A time series approach for clustering mass spectrometry data. Journal of Computational Science. 2012;3(5):344–355.

[40] Košmelj K, Batagelj V. Cross-sectional approach for clustering time varying data. Journal of Classification. 1990;7(1):99–109.

[41] Iglesias F, Kastner W. Analysis of similarity measures in times series clustering for the discovery of building energy patterns. Energies.2013;6(2): 579–597.

[42] Fu Tc, Chung Fl, Ng V, Luk R. Pattern discovery from stock time series using self-organizing maps. In: Workshop Notes of KDD2001 Workshop on Temporal Data Mining; 2001. p. 26–29.

[43] Aghabozorgi S, Teh YW. Stock market co-movement assessment using a three-phase clustering method. Expert Systems with Applications.2014;41(4): 1301–1314.

[44] Montero P, Vilar JA, et al. TSclust: An R package for time series clustering. Journal of Statistical Software. 2014;62 (1):1–43.

[45] Sardá-Espinosa A. Comparing time-series clustering algorithms in r using the dtwclust package. R package vignette. 2017;12:41.

[46] Fajer M, Meng Y, Roux B. The activation of c-Src tyrosine kinase: conformational transition pathway and free energy landscape. The Journal of Physical Chemistry B. 2017;121(15): 3352–3363.

Chapter 5

Importance of Protein Kinase and Its Inhibitor: A Review

Panneerselvam Theivendren, Selvaraj Kunjiappan, Yashoda Mariappa Hegde, Sivakumar Vellaichamy, Murugananthan Gopal, Senthil Rajan Dhramalingam and Sattanathan Kumar

Abstract

Deregulation of a broad range of protein kinases has been linked to the development and growth of cancer cells. Protein kinases are intracellular enzymes that regulate cell growth and proliferation as well as the triggering and regulation of immune responses. Protein kinases are important therapeutic targets in cancer because of their critical role in signalling mechanisms that drive malignant cell characteristics. Intensive efforts in drug research have been made in this area over the last two decades. The current study delves into the catalytic domain of a protein kinase as well as information transfer from the cell's membrane to internal targets. It also discusses the function of protein kinases in signal transduction and their cellular signalling pathways. Furthermore, it specifically outlines a systematic method to hybrid therapies to solve the issue of protein kinase resistance. The therapeutic use of nitric oxide, as well as other targets such as Phosphoinositide 3-kinases (PI3K), Protein Kinase B (Akt), serine/threonine protein kinase (mTOR), p38 mitogen-activated protein kinases (p38 MAPK), vascular endothelial growth factor receptors (VEGFR), epidermal growth factor receptors (EGFR), and anaplastic lymphoma (ALK) etc., According to the review article, selective therapy has shown high effectiveness in the treatment of advanced cancer, with protein kinase inhibitors being a main focus of the therapy. As a result, the latest review summarized that, the current state of science with the aim of identifying a novel protein kinase inhibitor that may be utilized in the treatment of advanced cancers.

Keywords: Protein kinases, Signal Transduction, Cellular signalling pathways, NO and Anticancer

1. Introduction

The protein kinase enzyme family has been one of the most significant drug targets in the 21st century due to the dysregulation of protein kinase function in several diseases, including cancer. Protein kinases assume a crucial role in the intracellular transduction on account of their capability to phosphorylate plenty of proteins. In recent years, various protein kinase inhibitors have been recognized and are being utilized effectively in the clinical sector. In 2020, the FDA approved the following medications for the treatment of the diseases listed: gastrointestinal stromal tumors), Capmatinib (non-small cell lung cancer), Pemigatinib (cholangiocarcinoma), Pralsetinib and Selpercatinib (non-small cell lung cancer, medullary thyroid cancer, and distinguished thyroid cancer), Selumetinib (neurofibromatosis type I), and Tucatinib (neurofibromatosis type I) (HER2-positive breast cancer). About every part of cellular activity is implicated in protein kinases [1]. It controls the metabolism, cell division and motion, movement, as well as immune and nervous system function and programmed cell death. The transfer of -phosphate from ATP to its protein substrates is catalyzed by protein kinase [2]. Protein kinase is a high-energy phosphate donor enzyme that donates a phosphate to other proteins. Phosphorylation is the process of converting one substance into another. In the reaction below, the substratum receives a group of phosphates and a phosphate group is donated by the high-energy ATP molecule. Trans-esterification results in a phosphorylated substrate; dephosphorylation is generated if the phosphoryphorylated substrate donates a phosphate group, and the phosphorylated substrate is grouped with ADP [3]. Protein kinases catalyze the following reaction:

$$\mathrm{MgATPl^{-} + Protein^{-}OH \rightarrow Protein^{-}O{:}PO32\_ + MgADP + H^{+}}$$

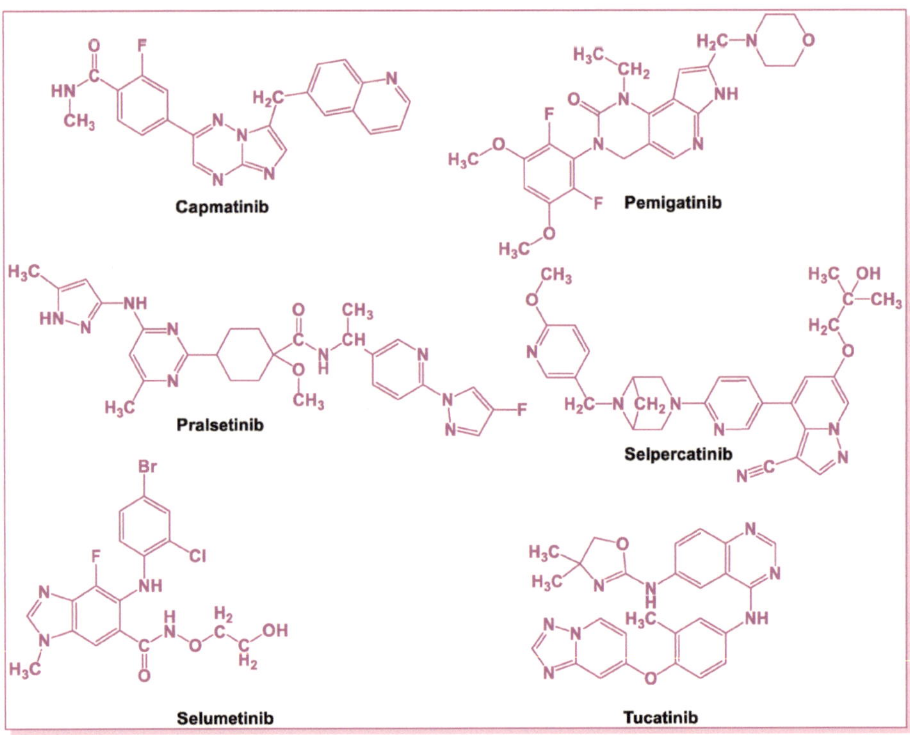

The human genome contains about 500 protein kinase genes, representing approximately 2% of all human genes [3]. Tyrosine kinases phosphorylate tyrosine hydroxyl groups in their targets, while serine/threonine kinases phosphorylate serine and threonine hydroxyl groups in their targets [4]. Protein kinases can be present in bacteria as well as plants. The majority of cellular pathways, especially those involved in signal transduction, are known to be regulated by kinases, and their actions can alter up to 30% of all human proteins. Protein kinases are enzymes that phosphorylate serine, threonine, tyrosine, or histidine residues in proteins. Phosphorylation can affect the role of a protein in a number of ways. It has the ability to alter the function of a protein, stabilise or kill it, localise it in a particular cellular compartment, and start or stop its association with other proteins. Protein kinases make up the majority of kinases which have had a lot of criticism. Phosphatases are involved in the regulation of proteins and enzymes, as well as cell signalling. Aside from allosteric regulation, the potential to affect protein behaviour is tremendous [3], and there are many methods for covalently altering a protein. Allosteric regulation evolved to react to signals from inside the cell, while phosphorylation evolved to respond to signals from outside the cell, according to Edwin Krebs' Hopkins Memorial Lecture. The fact that eukaryotic cells phosphorylate proteins even more frequently than prokaryotic cells supports this theory, implying that the more complicated cell form has evolved to react to a broader spectrum of signals [5]. The chemical feature of a kinase is to covalently attach an ATP phosphate group to one of three amino acids with a free hydroxyl group. While most kinases bind to serine and threonine, some (dual-specificity kinases) often bind to serine and tyrosine [3]. Protein kinases use two types of interactions to identify their physiological substrates in cells: (i) the active protein kinase site recognises the consensus phosphorylation sequence in the protein substratum, and (ii) distal interactions between the kinase and the substratum are mediated by binding a docking motif spastically isolated from the phosphorylation site in the substratum to a substratum. Protein kinases use these interactions to identify their protein substrates with extreme precision. The identification of possible protein kinase physiological substrates should be aided by understanding the molecular basis for these interactions. Since protein phosphorylation is so important, researchers have spent a lot of time trying to figure out how protein kinase signal transduction mechanisms work. Dysregulation of protein kinases is seen in a wide range of illnesses, including cancer and inflammatory conditions.

2. Importance of protein kinase's

Protein kinases are intracellular enzymes that regulate cell growth and proliferation as well as immune response triggering and control. Protein kinases are phosphotransferases that binds phosphate to the side chains of serine, threonine, or tyrosine residues in cells to phosphorylate them. Kinases are needed in the first phase of intracellular immune cell signalling. Kinases, for instance, bind to the intracellular component of receptors on T and B lymphocytes' cell surfaces, and once these receptors are engaged with their extracellular ligands, they trigger intracellular signalling cascades within these cells. Phosphate (P) is transferred from ATP to a serine, threonine, or tyrosine residue in protein by protein kinases (**Figure 1**). Phosphorylation acts as a'molecular shift,' enabling proteins to be triggered or deactivated directly. Protein phosphatases, on the other side, catalyze the elimination of the -phosphate from the target protein, which inhibits kinase function and reverses phosphorylation results [1, 3]. Serine (Ser or S), threonine (Thr or T), and tyrosine (Tyr or Y) residues account for more than one third of all protein phosphorylation events (O-phosphorylation) [3]. Just 1.8 per cent of tyrosine residues are phosphorylated, compared to 86.4 per cent of serine residues, 11.8 per cent of threonine residues, and 11.8 per cent of tyrosine residues [3, 4]. Tyrosine phosphorylation is peculiar among post-transitional modifications (PTM) in the EGFR band, including a tyrosine kinase domain. Histidine (His or H) and aspartate (Asp or D) metabolites may also be N-phosphorylated, but this process is less robust

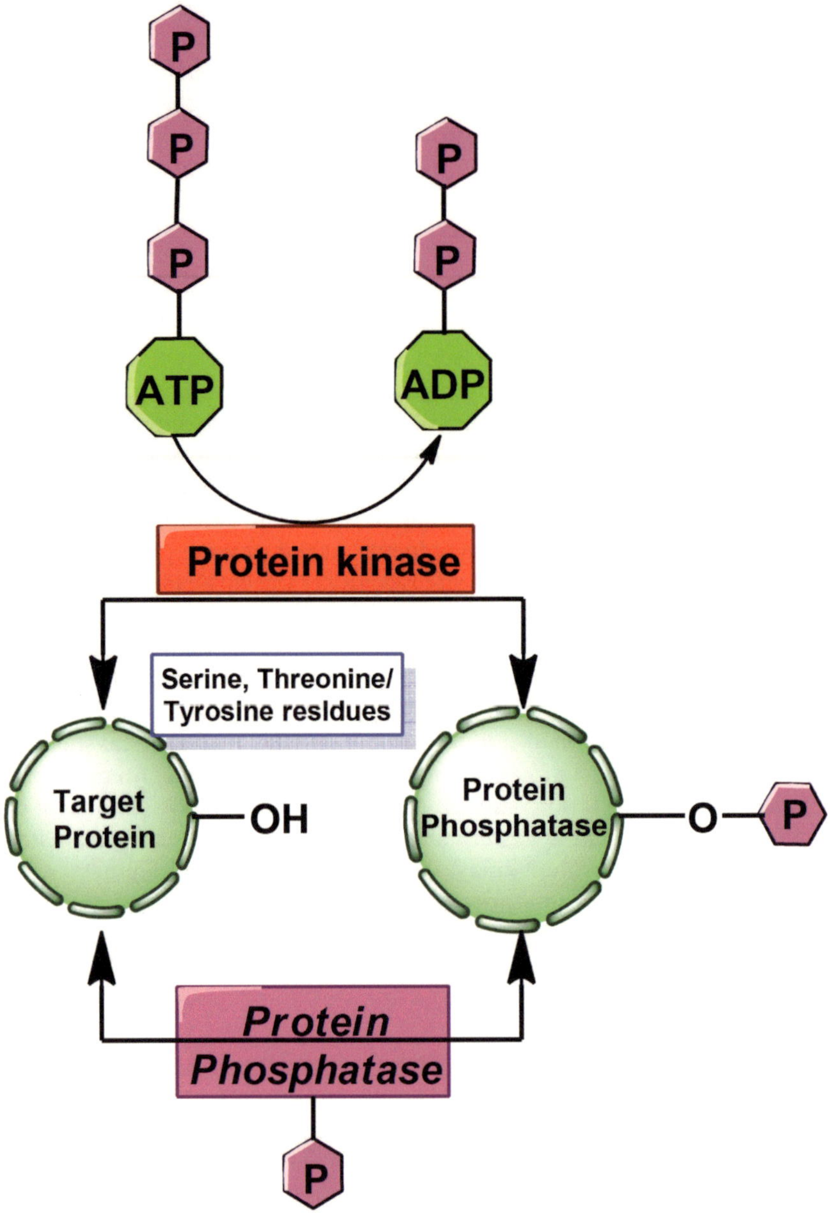

Figure 1.
Phosphorylation by protein kinase.

than other phosphorylation approaches. Since phosphorylation/dephosphorylation events mediated by different kinases and phosphatases trigger and deactivate several enzymes and receptors, protein phosphorylation is a central regulating mechanism in several cellular processes, including protein synthesis, cell division, signal transduction, cell forming, development, and ageing. In addition, the human genome contains 568 protein kinases and 156 protein phosphatases, both of which control phosphorylation events and thus play a key role in biological processes such as proliferation, differentiation, and apoptosis. Phosphorylation stimulates the p53 receptor, which stops gene replication, stops the cell cycle, starts DNA repair, and, in certain instances, helps the cell die [2]. Chronic inactivation of the p53 protein due to excess in the phosphorylation/dephosphorylation pathway will turn a cell cancerous. The 568 human protein kinases are classified based on the amino acid residues that they phosphorylate. The majority of kinases (serine/threonine kinases, or STKs) operate on both serine and threonine, while others (tyrosine kinases, or TKs) only work on one of the three amino acids (dual-specificity kinases; DSKs) [2]. STKs and TKs can be phosphorylated by the latter [6], with STKs accounting for about a quarter of all human protein kinases [2, 7]. STKs phosphorylate serine or threonine's OH group. DNA injury, as well as chemical signals like Ca2+/calmodulin, cyclic adenosine monophosphate/cyclic guanosine monophosphate (cAMP/cGMP), and diacylglycerol [8–16], trigger them. Protein kinase phosphorylation sets off a chain reaction that results in the phosphorylation of various amino acids [17]. Kinases may be programmed or deactivated in a variety of ways, including cis- or autophosphorylation, binding with activator or inhibitor proteins, or checking their localization in the cell with a substrate [3].

3. Catalytic domain of a protein kinase

The catalytic domain of a protein kinase is divided into two parts: N-terminal and C-terminal. A peptidic strand connects the two, forming an active site with a front pocket (catalytic residues) and a back pocket. A stored lysine residue and a residue "gatekeeper" control access to the back pocket. The catalytic domain is unavailable while activated since the propellers of the N- and C-terminal sub domains move inward. Non-catalytic domains of the kinases allow substrate attachment and signalling protein recruitment [3]. Kinases have gained in popularity in recent years, thanks to their functions in signal transduction and amplitude modulation, as well as their importance in signalling [18–20]. Many databases have been created to aid in the analysis of phospho-signalling networks [21, 22]. According to a review, protein kinases have been linked to over 400 diseases, either directly or indirectly. As a consequence, protein kinases are regarded as one of the most significant drug targets. Small molecular compounds that inhibit protein phosphorylation and thus resist activation can be used to target kinases. These small molecule inhibitors reduce kinase gene expression by disrupting ATP-kinase binding, intervening with kinase-protein interactions, and disrupting ATP-kinase binding. Protein kinase targets (SYK) include Janus kinase (JAK), mitogen-activated protein kinase (MAPK), and spleen tyrosine kinase [1–3].

4. Manifestation of signal transduction

The transmission of information from the cell's membrane to internal targets (within the cell) initiates a chain of molecular events that culminate in a biological response to the affector molecule (**Figure 2**). Advances in biochemical and molecular biological techniques have enabled the discovery of essential enzymes involved in the transduction phase, as well as the production of several natural and synthetic modulators of biological processes, over the last decade [5, 23]. Researchers have better understood molecular events in both natural and pathological settings because of these techniques. As new information regarding molecular interactions that regulate cellular responses has become accessible, the potential for designing and creating new drugs to cure cancer, central nervous system disorders (Alzheimer's disease), cardiovascular disorders (hypertension), skin disorders (inflammation), diabetes mellitus, and other chronic diseases has grown.

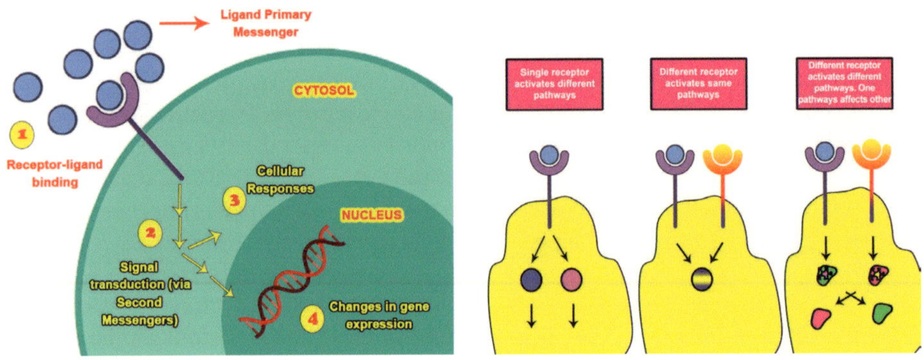

Figure 2.
The event of signal transduction.

5. Protein kinase's role in signal transduction

Second messengers such as cyclic AMP (adenosine monophosphate) and calcium are needed for the majority of isozymes to act [24, 25]. Kinases and phosphatases are known as "third messengers" because of this. Signal transduction is the process by which an extracellular primary signal is converted into an intracellular second messenger. In ligand-gated (ion channel) receptors, ion influx serves as a second messenger. G-protein-linked receptors can stimulate not only a second, but also a third and fourth messenger while they are activated. The ultimate endpoint could be the manipulation of gene transcription to generate messenger RNA (mRNA) and then mRNA translation to produce a protein specific to that gene. When a receptor attaches to a signalling molecule, it activates a signal transduction process. The four forms of messenger systems are as follows:

The first messengers are G-protein-linked messengers, kinases, and phosphatases, followed by phospho-calcium/cyclic AMP response element-binding (CREB) protein as the fourth messenger.

6. Protein kinase's role in cellular signalling pathways

Protein kinases play a number of roles in the body [26, 27]. Protein kinases are involved in variety of cellular signalling pathways **Figure 3** (phosphorylation). Protein kinases have different physiological functions in various systems, such as the cardiovascular system [27]. Troponin is triggered when PKA is activated, increasing the binding of excitation contractions. It also increases the contractility of the heart muscle. PKC activation phosphorylates other proteins in smooth muscles, despite the fact that cytosolic Ca++ combines with calmodulin (CAM) to activate myosin light chain kinase, causing smooth muscle contraction [25, 28]. Protein kinase A causes an increase in membrane water permeability by increasing the rate of exocytosis of water-containing vesicles (WCVs) into the apical membrane and decreasing the rate of endocytosis of WCVs from the apical membrane in the kidneys. The mitogen-activated protein (MAP) kinase pathway is activated by angiotensin I receptors (At1) in the kidney, which promotes cell development, especially in vascular and cardiac cells. It raises proton changes, particularly C-fos and C-jun, which regulate the transcription of several genes involved in cell growth [23]. At1 activates Protein Kinase A, which causes phosphorylation of proteins involved in aldosterone synthesis, neurotransmission facilitation, CNS outcomes, and renal impact.

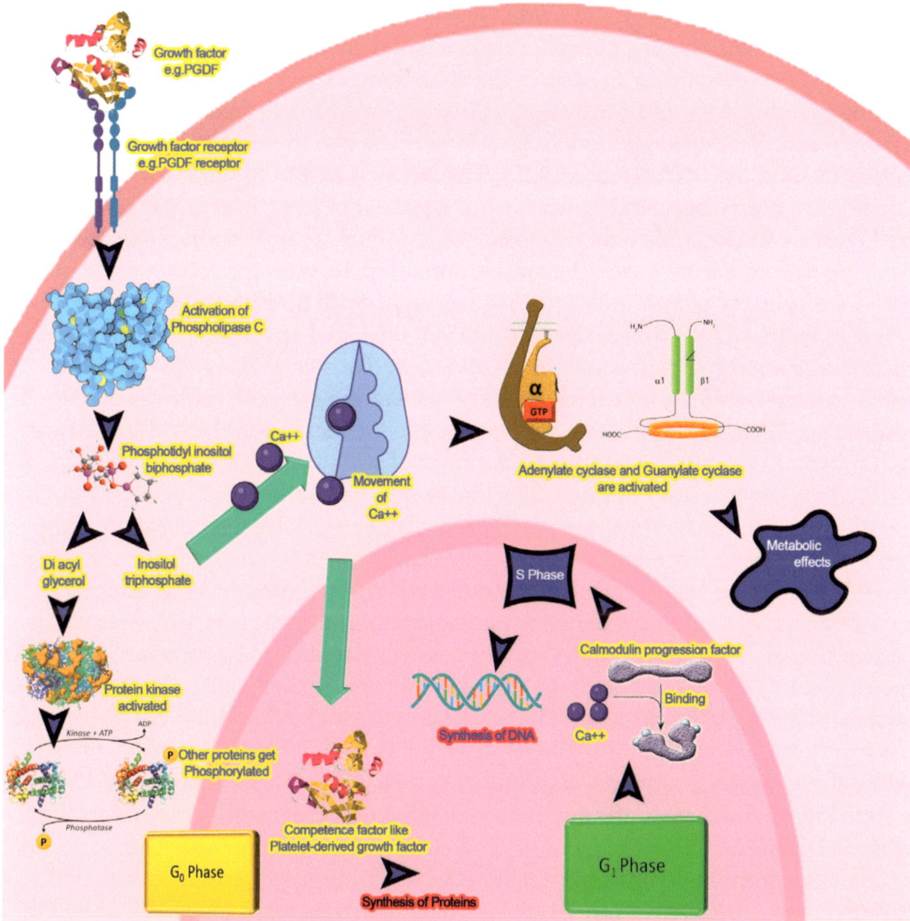

Figure 3.
The protein kinase sequence of signaling process.

7. A review of functions of protein kinases

Protein kinases assign a phosphate group from the ATP gamma location to specific amino acid residues in proteins and peptides. Protein phosphorylation is implicated in a variety of physiological processes, including glucose absorption, signalling, epigenetic modifications, and cell cycle progression. Diabetes, cardiovascular disease, Alzheimer's disease, and cancer, to name a few illnesses, have all been linked to phosphorylation deficiencies. Monitoring protein kinase activity is crucial for better understanding disease molecular mechanisms and determining whether or not a treatment is successful. Inhibiting pathological phosphorylation can aid in the treatment of these diseases as well [29]. The desire to solve the three-dimensional structures of many of these enzymes sparked interest in academia and the pharmaceutical industry due to these factors [30]. According to Steinberg SF, cyclin-dependent kinases (CDKs) are a form of serine/threonine kinase whose activity is mediated by cyclin, a protein regulatory subunit. Eukaryotic cell division and transcription are aided by CDKs. PKC is a serine/threonine kinase that regulates a variety of natural cellular responses and also plays a role in the pathogenesis of ischemia–reperfusion injury. The Abelson murine leukaemia virus (Abl) proto-oncogene is a non-receptor tyrosine kinase that is activated by both extrinsic ligands such as growth factor receptors and intrinsic signals such as DNA damage and oxidative stress. c-Abl shuttles between the cytosolic and nuclear compartments, phosphorylates a variety of cellular substrates (including adaptor proteins, other kinases, cytoskeletal proteins, transcription factors, and chromatin modifiers), and controls signalling pathways implicated in actin polymerization and cytoskeletal remodelling, cell adhesion and motility, transcriptional regulation, and the DNA structure [30]. The mitogen-activated protein kinase 4 (MKK4) has been discovered to be a central regulator of liver regeneration, according to Klövekorn P et al., and could be a valuable drug goal for treating liver diseases by restoring the organ's intrinsic regenerative potential. According to Wüstefeld et al., MKK4 is a primary promotor for liver regeneration, with positive results on hepatocyte regeneration, robustness, fibrosis, and Fas-mediated apoptosis [31]. The primary intracellular energy sensor, according to Jovanovic-Tucovic et al., is AMP-activated protein kinase (AMPK), which triggers ATP-generating catabolic pathways while inhibiting ATP-requiring processes in response to the increase in the AMP/ATP ratio and/or oxidative stress. Depending on the form of stimuli and the intensity/length of AMPK activation, this serine/threonine kinase may be neuroprotective or neurotoxic, and its dysregulation has been attributed to neurodegenerative disorders including Parkinson's disease. Serine/threonine-protein kinase B/Akt is another crucial protein kinase for neuronal cell metabolism and survival. Phosphodiesterase 5A inhibitors, such as Sildenafil, have been shown to protect against ischemic injury by decreasing cardiac Na+/H+ exchanger (NHE1) activity, which is regulated by protein kinase G, as mentioned by Diaz RG et al. [32]. In 1954, Burnett and Kennedy discovered the Casein Kinase 2 (CK2) catalyst. It's a Ser/Thr protein kinase that's acidophilic and pleiotropic, and it's crucial for cell viability. When coupled with CK1, it acts as a catalyst, phosphorylating Casein protein in vitro (but not in vivo) [32]. The use of enacted AMP protein kinase as a therapeutic target for ischemia–reperfusion injury was identified by Rong Ding et al. [33].

The most popular drug targets include BCR-Abl, B-Raf, vascular endothelial growth factor receptors (VEGFR), epidermal growth factor receptors (EGFR), and ALK. The bulk of small molecule protein kinase antagonists adhere to the protein kinase domain and treat cancers such as myelofibrosis, polycythemiavera, persistent immune thrombocytopenia, rheumatoid arthritis, idiopathic pulmonary fibrosis, and glaucoma [34].

Human eukaryotic protein kinases (ePKs) have been divided into nine classes, according to Gaji et al. The following are examples of these: (1) the AGC group, which includes PKA, PKB (At1, At2, At3) PKG, and PKC; (2) the Ca^{2+}/calmodulin-dependent protein kinase (CAMK) group, which includes calcium/calmodulin-dependent protein kinases (CAMK) and mitogen activated protein kinase activating protein kinases (MAPKAPKs); (3) the casein kinase 1 (CK1) group, which has 12 members; (4) the CMGC group, which has 6161members including cyclin-dependent protein kinases (CDK), mitogen-activated protein kinases (MAPK), glycogen synthase kinase (GSK) and cyclin dependent kinase like (CDKL) families; (5) The STE group (related to yeast non-mating or sterile genes) has 47 members who are MAPK upstream regulators; (6) the tyrosine kinase (TK) group has 90 members, including 58 receptor protein kinases (RTKs) and 32 non-receptor tyrosine kinases; (7) the tyrosine kinase like (TKL) group has 43 members, and proteins in this family; (8) the receptor guanylylcyclase (RGC) group consists of five members; and (9) the 'other' group has 83 members. In addition, 40 kinases are known as atypical kinases, one of which is the mitochondrial pyruvate dehydrogenase kinase [35]. For types and classes of protein kinases refer **Tables 1** and **2**. AMP-activated protein kinase (AMPK) senses energy levels and controls metabolic processes to maintain homeostasis. The function of AMPK is influenced by the supply of nutrients such as carbohydrates, lipids, and amino acids. AMPK function is impaired by overnutrition,

Types	Examples	Functions
Serine/threonine-specific protein kinases	Calcium/calmodulin-dependent protein kinase II (CaMKII)	Phosphorylate serine or threonine's –OH (hydroxyl) functional group.
Tyrosine-specific protein kinases	Platelet derived growth factor (PDGF) receptor Epidermal growth factor (EGF) receptor1 Insulin growth factor (IGF1) receptor Stem cell factor (scf) receptor	Processes alzheimer's amyloid precursor protein, epithelial cell migration and carcinoma invasion, spermatogonia osmoregulation, and antiaging survival factor
Histidine-specific protein kinases	Histidine kinase	The histidine kinase family is structurally similar to the pyruvate dehydrogenase family of kinases in animals.
Mixed kinases	Muscle action potential kinase (MAPK)	Involved in the cascade of muscle action potential kinase

Table 1.
A summary the types of protein kinases based on amino acid residue.

Types	Functions			
Protein kinase A (PKA)	Acts as a catalyst, allowing intracellular proteins to be catalysed. Glycogen, sugar, and lipid metabolism are all regulated by this protein. Phosphorylate acetyl-CoA carboxylase and pyruvate dehydrogenase in adipocytes, myocytes, and hepatocytes, resulting in acetyl-CoA-lipogenesis. The dopamine signal is translated into cells in the nucleus acumens neurons.			
Protein kinase B (PKB)	Akt	Akt1	Akt2	Akt3
	Cell proliferation, apoptosis, transcription, and cell migration are all involved in glucose metabolism. Cell survival - both actively and indirectly facilitate growth factor-mediated cell survival. Glycogen synthesis is aided by metabolism. Angiogenesis is linked to tumour growth and angiogenesis.	Is implicated in: cellular survival pathways, by inhibiting apoptosis processes. skeletal muscle hypertrophy and general tissue growth. the transforming retrovirus as the oncogene	The insulin signalling pathway has been linked to this protein. Glucose transport induction is a term used to describe the process of causing glucose	It tends to be expressed primarily in the brain. The brains of mice lacking Akt 3 are weak.
Protein kinase C (PKC)	Phosphorylation of intracellular proteins is catalysed by this enzyme, which changes their activities. Controls cellular growth and differentiation.			

Table 2.
Summary of classes of protein kinases [34].

inflammation, and hypersecretion of certain anabolic hormones, such as insulin, which is exacerbated by food shortages and inhibited by obesity. According to Zhao and Saltiel, activating AMPK in the liver inhibits de novo lipogenesis, promoting fatty acid oxidation (β -oxidation). Furthermore, AMPK activation prevents hepatic steatosis by inhibiting the production of free fatty acids from adipose tissue (**Figure 4**) [36]. On the other side, Alghamdi et al. investigated the function of

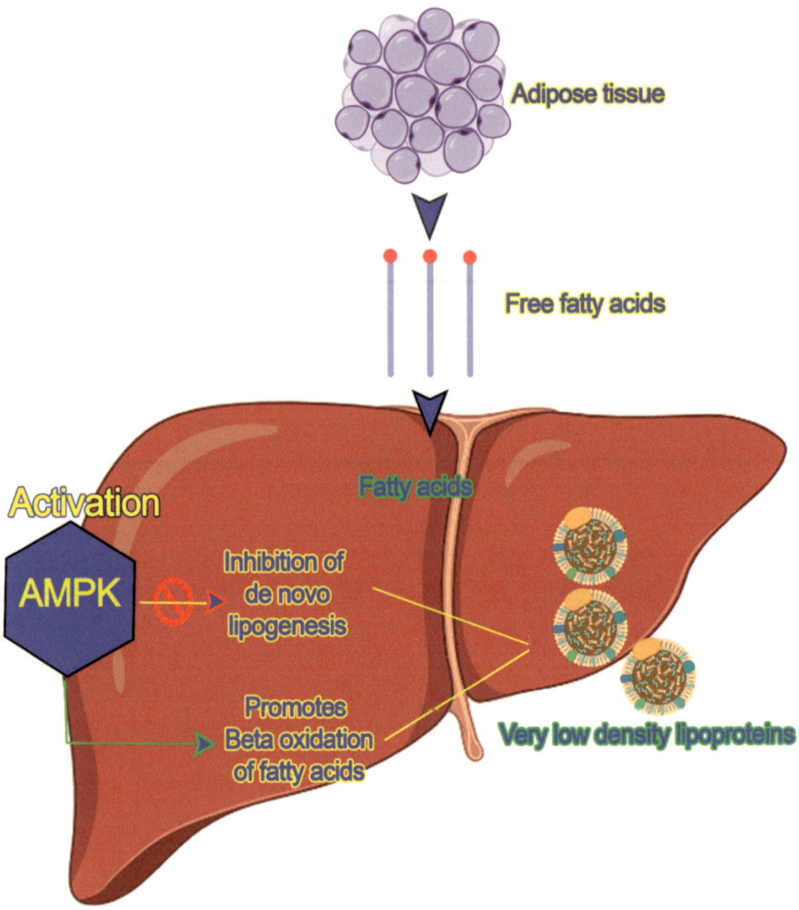

Figure 4.
Regulation of hepatic steatosis by AMPK.

AMPK in nutrient absorption by tissues, especially glucose and fatty acid uptake. Because of its impact on carbohydrate and lipid metabolism, rising FA oxidation and decreasing lipogenesis, AMPK activation has been proposed as a therapeutic goal for nutrient overload. In NAFLD/NASH (non-alcoholic fatty liver disease/non-alcoholic steatohepatitis), nutrient overload induces hepatic steatosis, which leads to fibrosis and liver injury. Hepatic steatosis is the accumulation of ectopic lipids in the liver and is closely linked to obesity, insulin resistance and type-2-diabetes.

De novolipogenesis (DNL) from carbohydrates or increased FA absorption and triglyceride synthesis cause lipid accumulation in the liver. Increased hepatic FA oxidation, on the other hand, reduces steatosis [37]. Li et al. results suggest that AMPK may be used as a clinical therapy for the treatment of cholestatic liver damage. The ability to evaluate the dose- and time-effects of AMPK activation in various models representing various stages of cholestatic liver injury is critical not just for determining the efficacy of AMPK as a targeted therapy for treating cholestatic liver injury, but also for providing crucial scientific proof for clinical practice and translational studies of existing AMPK inducers [38].

In recent pharmacological study, protein kinases have become one of the most widely researched therapeutic targets, especially in cancer and inflammation studies. For the treatment of cancer and inflammation, the US Food and Drug Administration has licenced 32 small-molecule protein kinase inhibitors. However, no medication successfully treats neuroinflammation and/or neurodegenerative conditions due to a lack of protein kinase drug targets for CNS disorders. According to new findings, some protein kinases have recently been established as promising drug targets in the treatment of neuroinflammation and/or neurodegenerative diseases. Lee and Suk investigated a number of protein kinases that are increasingly being seen as potential therapies in microglia-mediated neuroinflammation (**Figure 5**). Because of their critical roles in neuronal toxicity, some of these kinases, such as LRRK2, MST1, and tyrosine kinases (c-Abl, Src, and Fyn), have been proposed as potential drug targets, while others were presented here as novel protein kinase drug candidates because of their critical roles in microglial activation [39]. Many neurodegenerative disorders, such as Parkinson's disease (PD), Alzheimer's disease (AD), and stroke, are due to microglia-mediated neuroinflammation. Microglia-mediated neuroinflammation has been compared to protein kinases such as leucine-rich repeat kinase 2 (LRRK2) and mammalian Ste20-like kinase 1 (MST1), Src family protein tyrosine kinases (SFKs), a cellular homolog of the Abelson murine leukaemia virus oncogene (c-Abl), and TAM family receptor tyros TLRs, TNFR, CD11b, and P2Y12 protein kinases are all known to play a role in microglial activation by relaying signals from different exogenous inducers through cell surface receptors. Parkinson's disease and Alzheimer's disease all have protein aggregates as a pathological function (a-synuclein [a-SYN] in PD and Ab peptides in AD). These protein aggregates bind to TLR, CD11b, and other microglial receptors, triggering a number of intracellular signalling pathways. They are activated as a consequence of neuronal death or other proliferation mechanisms. Bacterial lipopolysaccharide (LPS), adenosine diphosphate (ADP), tumour necrosis factor (TNF), and RNA

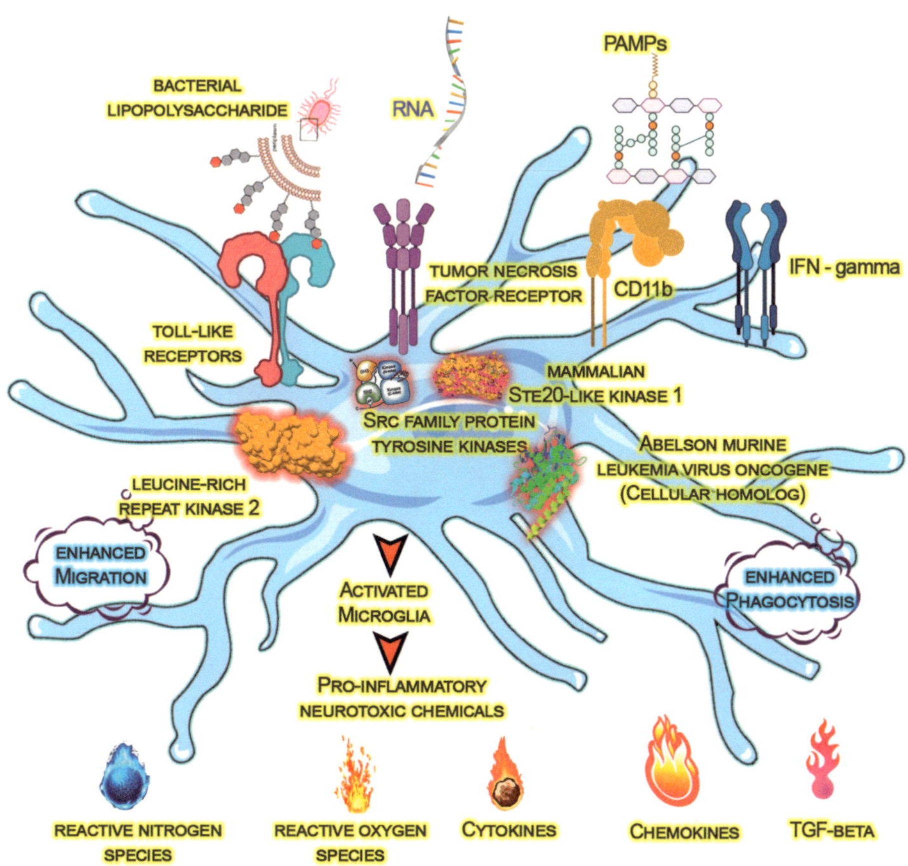

Figure 5.
Microglia-mediated neuroinflammation.

virus are among the other triggers that activate microglia through TLRs, P2Y12, and TNFR. TAM receptor tyrosine kinases including Axl and Mer are involved in several areas of microglia-mediated neuroinflammatory pathology in PD. As a consequence of their activation, activated microglia produce a broad variety of proinflammatory cytokines, chemokines, and reactive oxygen/nitrogen species (ROS/RNS). In response to stimuli and intracellular protein kinases, activated microglia increased migration and phagocytic action. Several studies have linked protein kinases to neuronal toxicity and microglial activation. In comparison to neurons, only a few protein kinases (PKs) have arisen as critical signalling components modulating microglial activation. Some kinases, such as Leucine-rich repeat kinase 2 (LRRK2), mammalian Ste20-like kinase 1 (MST1), tyrosine kinases, and mitogen-activated protein kinases (MAPKs), tend to be involved in both neuronal toxicity and microglial activation, while TAM receptor tyrosine kinases (RTKs) like Axl and Mer also recently emerged as new targeted therapies for inflammation caused by microglia [39].

According to Simon Diering et al., the modulation of the b1-adrenoreceptor (AR) signalling pathway regulates the contraction and relaxation of the heart by activating cAMP-dependent protein kinase (PKA) and subsequent cardiac protein phosphorylation. The key cardiac protein phosphatases, PP2A and PP1, prevent phosphorylation. Intra molecular disulfide formation in the catalytic subunits of

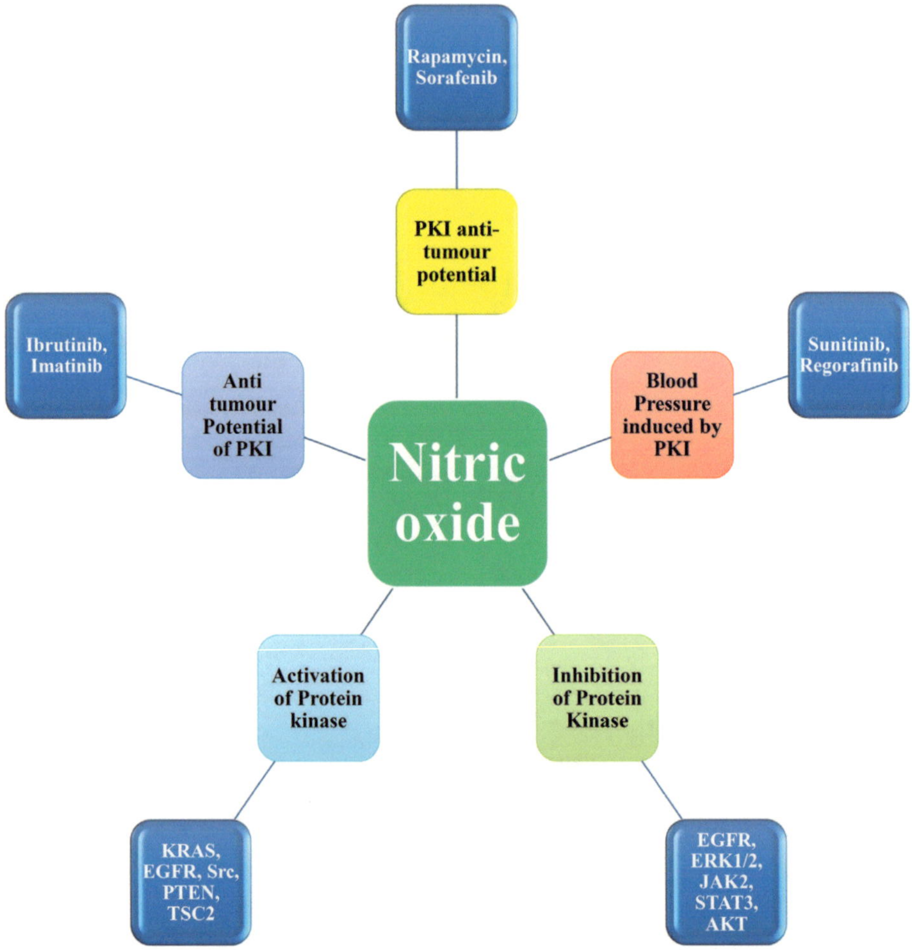

Figure 6.
Impact of NO on protein kinases and PKIs activities.

both kinases and phosphatases inhibits their function [40]. Hashemol hossein discovered that CK2 is involved in a number of phases in the biology of striated skeletal muscle, including myogenesis and homeostasis in adult muscle, as well as neuromuscular junctions, which connect muscle fibres and motor nerves. CK2 regulates protein import in myotube organelles, as well as the consistency and dignity of the postsynaptic machinery in neuromuscular junctions and the muscular cytoskeleton [40]. It's also becoming clear that CK2's function in processes that dynamically regulate the phosphoproteome of muscle cells is significant, and that it's likely to play a role in maintaining muscle homeostasis at the molecular level.

A wide range of protein kinase inhibitors (PKIs) have entered various stages of clinical development in the last two decades, with various properties and potential applications, such as different selectivity and modes of binding to kinases, and some have been licenced by the FDA. PKIs have therefore developed themselves as a significant class of cancer medicines, and their therapeutic ability continues to attract attention. In fact, studying kinase biology in relation to PKI development is an essential part of targeted therapies. The resistance of cancer cells to PKI therapies necessitates the development of new therapeutic options. As a result, new generation PKIs have been built and tested in the hopes of overcoming resistance. According to Ghione et al., NO may directly or indirectly regulate protein kinases involved in essential cancer signalling pathways, as seen with PKIs. The NO donor NTG has been studied in a growing number of clinical trials as an anticancer treatment when combined with radiotherapy or chemotherapy.

NO's ambivalent impact on PKI (encouraging or inhibiting PKI's anticancer potential) and the action of protein kinases are summarised (regulated at the transcriptional or the post-translational level by NO) **Figure 6** [41].

8. NO acts as a kinase activator

According to several reports, the intracellular production of NO by NOS is needed for the phosphorylation and subsequent activation of EGFR signalling pathways. Overexpression of iNOS in a number of tumours, including breast cancer, has been related to tumour development and angiogenesis. Indeed, high iNOS expression has been linked to EGFR phosphorylation, activation, and poor prognosis in various breast cancer subtypes.

9. NO acts as a kinase inhibitor

NO has been shown to have a detrimental regulatory impact on protein kinases in many experiments, which is compatible with its unclear role in cancer. By inhibiting the activity of many protein kinases, NO may inhibit pathways implicated in cancer cell proliferation and survival. For some of these protein kinases, selective protein kinase inhibitors (PKIs) are currently being investigated [41].

Mori et al. investigated whether the biguanide anti-hyperglycemic medication metformin dilates retinal blood vessels in rats. *In vivo*, photographs of the ocular fundus were taken with a high-resolution optical fundus camera, and the diameters of retinal blood vessels were determined. The pulse rate and systemic blood pressure were also constantly monitored. Metformin (0.01–0.3 mg/kg/min) raised the diameters of retinal blood vessels in a dose-dependent way. Metformin's retinal vasodilator effect was blocked by compounds, an AMPK inhibitor, and NG-nitro-L-arginine methyl ester, a nitric oxide (NO) synthase inhibitor. The AMPK activator

5-aminoimidazole-4-carboxamide-1-D-ribonucleoside (AICAR, 0.01–1 mg/kg/min) generated similar effects. The effects of metformin and AICAR on mean blood pressure and heart rate were not important. When NO synthase was inhibited, however, a significant presser reaction to AICAR was observed. These findings indicate that metformin activates AMPK, which dilates retinal blood vessels, and that NO plays a significant role in the retinal vasodilator reaction after AMPK activation (**Figure 7**). According to this report, the anti-diabetic medication metformin dilates retinal blood vessels by activating AMPK, which is the first pharmacological proof according to this report. Metformin inhibits inflammatory reactions and angiogenesis in the retina, in addition to lowering blood glucose levels. Aside from these benefits, the retinal vasodilator influence can help prevent or delay the development of diabetic retinopathy [42]. KN-93, a calmodulin-dependent protein kinase inhibitor, prevents neuronal cell viability in an *in vitro* Alzheimer's disease model, according to Yilmaz. Alzheimer's disease is the most prevalent form of dementia in people over the age of 65, and it is marked by memory loss that progresses over time. The neurofibrillary tangles formed by hyperphosphorylated tau and the senile plaques generated by the -amyloid peptide (A 1–4) are the key cardinal lesions consistent with Alzheimer's disease. CaMKII, a central enzyme in memory development, incorporates transient knowledge reflecting both past and current cellular behaviour into the complex essence of "continuous" calcium signalling. Although the alpha and beta isoforms of the CaMKII enzyme have been shown to play a role in memory development, the role of the gamma and delta isoforms is yet to be determined [43]. Researchers have continued to design and create new Rho kinase inhibitors throughout the decade after Fasudil was approved in Japan for the

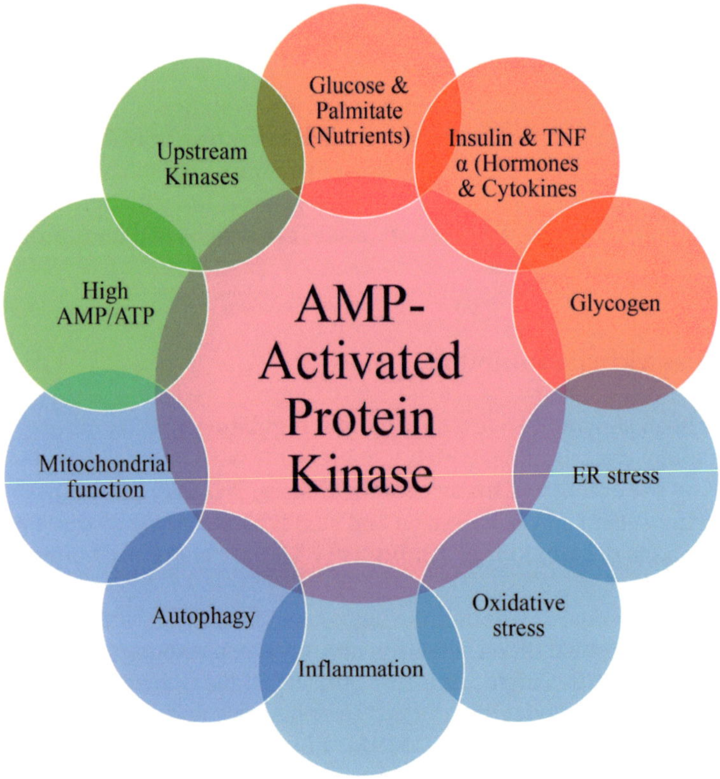

Figure 7.
AMPK activated protein kinase.

treatment and prevention of cerebral vasospasm and subarachnoid haemorrhage. Rho kinase inhibitors have been shown to be useful in the treatment of neurodegenerative conditions, coronary diseases, metabolic syndrome, and glaucoma. Both animal and human trials have supported the beneficial effect of Rho kinase inhibitors in the improvement of lung arterial relaxation and remodelling, suggesting that they may be useful in the treatment of pulmonary hypertension. According to Abedi et al., Rho kinase inhibitors have also been shown to be successful in the preventing and treating pulmonary fibrosis, with increasing confirmation that the Rho/ROCK signalling system is involved in actinomyosin contraction and actin filament assembly. Down regulation of the Rho/ROCK signalling system is aided by specific Rho kinase inhibitors. Rho induction has also been linked to other possible clinical uses. For example, statins' action on atherosclerosis has been linked to their Rho inhibitory effect, as has simvastatin's preventive role in chronic pulmonary hypertension. Inhibitions of RhoA activity and down regulation of Rho kinase activity are thought to be involved in ibuprofen's beneficial effects in ventilator-induced lung injury. In humans, the use of a Rho kinase inhibitor has not been confirmed to have severe hemodynamic side effects, and it has been shown to have excellent tolerability. Based on post-market monitoring, haemorrhage (1.7 percent) and hypotension were the most frequent adverse effects recorded for fasudil (0.07 percent). Rho kinase inhibitors' protection profile may be their most significant benefit in the care of acute lung inflammation acute lung inflammation (ALI). However, since these inhibitors are multifunctional, they seem to be more beneficial than any other medicinal agents utilised in the care of ALI. Rho kinase inhibitors have been shown to improve cell viability in several *in vitro* trials. In our search of the literature, we identified no single report that contrasted the effectiveness and/or risks of Rho kinase inhibitors to those of other therapeutic agents. Human evidence and clinical trials confirming the beneficial effects of Rho kinase inhibitors in ALI are minimal or non-supportive, despite preclinical studies endorsing the beneficial effects of Rho kinase inhibitors in ALI. For example, in the case of sepsis and inflammatory diseases, around 150 compounds reached clinical trials based on preclinical evidence, none of which were Rho kinase inhibitors, but failed to hit the market, indicating the need for improved preclinical efficacy protocols. Finally, it appears that up regulation of the RhoA/ROCK signalling pathway is essential in the pathogenesis of ALI.

Rho kinase inhibitors have shown in limited preclinical studies to have a high potential for preventing the development of ALI. Inflammation, immune cell migration, apoptosis, coagulation, contraction, and cell adhesion were all inhibited, which had positive effects.

Endothelium barrier impairment and edoema was reduced as a result of increased pulmonary endothelial cells. Inhibition of Rho kinase seems to be a successful new method for treating ALI [ARDS]. However, more clinical trials are needed to back up this hypothesis [44].

p38 MAP kinase inhibitors in signalling pathways as possible neuroprotective drugs were studied by Ahmed et al. The discovery of p38 MAP kinase's connection to TNF- and IL-1 synthesis in 1994 established the fact that the net biological effect of p38 activation is the downstream development of various inflammatory mediators that initiate the activation and recruitment of leukocytes. p38 MAP kinase signalling is linked to excitotoxicity (glutamine aggregation in synapses) in astrocytes, synaptic plasticity, and tau phosphorylation in neurons, and it leads to neuroinflammation. The activity of the p38 MAP kinase may play a role in the pathophysiology of a variety of neurodegenerative disorders, including Parkinson's disease (both hereditary and sporadic) and multiple sclerosis. There are four different isoforms of the p38 MAP kinase, all of which share roughly 60%

homology. The p38a MAP kinase is a major isoform of p38 that is activated under inflammatory conditions and is a key player in the synthesis of inflammatory mediators. Upstream MAP3Ks normally trigger downstream MAP kinases (MKK3 and MKK6). MKK3 and MKK6 trigger p38 MAPK through dual phosphorylation on Tyr182 and Thr180 once enabled. In neurodegenerative diseases, p38 MAP kinase may control hyperphosphorylation of Tau (PHFTau), leading to its dissociation from the cytoskeleton and self-aggregation. PHF-Tau is a significant component of the neurofibrillary tangles, which are one of the most common aberrant forms seen in Alzheimer's cases. In the astrocytoma cell line U373 MG, p38 MAP kinase mediates substance P (SP)-induced IL-6 expression independently of NF-B activation. SP caused p38 MAP kinase phosphorylation, which was independent of p42/44 MAPK and protein kinase C activation [45]. Gordon et al. found that stimulation of protein kinase c delta in response to neurotoxic stressors (a-synuclein, TNF-, LPS) plays a crucial role in the induction of dopaminergic neuronal failure. Protein kinase c delta deficiency was shown to reduce locomotor deficiencies and decrease proinflammatory reaction in the mouse substantianigra in an experimental model of Parkinson's disease. The function of p38 MAP kinase inhibitors in the treatment of neurodegenerative disorders has been investigated, with a particular emphasis on their regulatory pathways [46]. According to Lund et al., CEP-1347 inhibits cytokine synthesis in human or murine microglia primary cultures as well as monocyte or macrophage-derived cell lines stimulated with Ab140 or endotoxins. The MLK inhibitor CEP-1347 inhibited the activation of the cJun/JNK signalling pathways in stressed neurons.

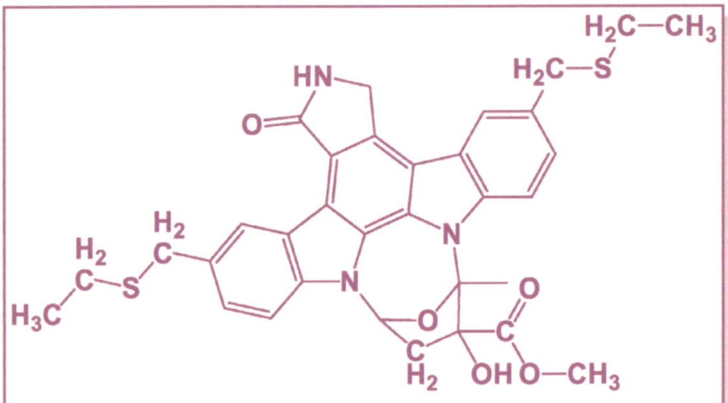

CEP 1347

In PD animal experiments, the inhibitor also reduced neurodegeneration. It is important to provide a thorough understanding of the signal transduction mechanisms involved in microglia-mediated inflammation in order to find therapies that can be used to cure neurological disorders. The p38 MAP kinase inhibitors and JNK signalling pathways specifically allow a better choice to be investigated further due to their potential to decrease proinflammatory cytokines production and their intracellular signalling pathway [47]. Watts et al., [48] and Wu et al., [49] recently published studies that say MAP4K4. According to Wu et al. [49], factors secreted in motor neuron cultures trigger MAP4K4.Following MAP4K4 activation, motor neurons die. As a result, MAP4K4 reduction will affect motor neuron viability through I attenuation of the c-Jun apoptotic pathway, and (ii) activation of autophagy mediated by FoxO1 that reduces protein aggregate accumulation and depicts that the activation of the p38 MAP kinase pathway in various cell types and pathways in neurodegenerative diseases.

10. Differential modulation of phosphorylation

In a single cell method, Basken et al. used phosphoproteomics to compare molecular responses to inhibitors that target protein kinases in several tiers of the MAPK cascade. They learned a lot regarding oncogenic BRAF signalling in melanoma cells, as well as new knowledge about MAPK pathway organisation, phosphorylation specificity, and off-target responses to therapeutics that are currently in use or being developed. The following results may be drawn from the study's findings:

First, there is a lot of variation between the phosphosites that are substantially influenced by MKK1/2 and ERK1/2 inhibitors. There were no answers that were specific to MKK1/2 or ERK1/2 inhibitors. This indicates that the signalling system is mostly absent of MKK1/2 targets that split upstream of ERK1/2. Comparing the BRAF inhibitor vemurafenib to the MKK1/2 inhibitor selumetinib in a previous analysis from our lab revealed identical results. The observed results suggest that signalling downstream of oncogenic BRAF requires a linear organisation of protein kinases, from BRAF to MKK1/2, and from MKK1/2 to ERK1/2, rather than a bifurcation in the pathway.

Second, the 161 sites controlled by all four MKK1/2 and ERK1/2 inhibitors revealed phosphorylation sites most likely to be bona fide targets of the MAPK pathway, allowing us to recognise phosphorylation sites most likely to be bona fide targets of the MAPK pathway. Moreover, hundreds of phosphosites have been identified as possible new ERK targets. Just 20% of the 103 phosphosites with Ser/Thr-Pro sequence specificity for ERK met existing ERK targets, implying 82 additional direct phosphorylation targets. A subset of 47 previously unreported phosphosites is prioritised as probable ERK1/2 substrates by searching for markers of MAPK substrates, such as proximity to Pro at position P-2 and the inclusion of DEF or DEJL docking motifs. The importance of this study is that, considering the fact that more than 700 ERK phosphorylation sites have been identified *in vitro* and/or *in vivo*, the amount of sites yet to be found is uncertain. The use of phosphoproteomics to find new substrates is hampered by a lack of understanding of kinase inhibitor specificity, as well as the risk of off-target results. Where a pathway signals linearly, as tends to be the case with the enzymes in the MAPK pathway, contrasting the coordinated effects of several inhibitors on more than one tier of the kinase cascade, as well as sequence determinants of ERK substrates, offers a rigorous filter for specificity. The findings indicate that ERK1/2 regulates new types of cellular processes, and they add for understanding of the pleiotropy of cellular responses that this important signalling kinase may influence.

Third, they discovered that 21 of the phosphosites observed to react to at least one of four kinase inhibitors only reacted to one of the four compounds, whilst the other three were obviously unresponsive. This serves as a useful filter for detecting inhibitor off-target results. Surprisingly, the majority of unambiguous off-target phosphosites reacted to the ERK1/2 inhibitor GDC0994, while responses to other kinase inhibitors were scarce. This is something to think about if you're looking at ERK1/2 inhibitors as a way to tackle resistance to BRAF and MKK1/2 inhibitor combinations. The inhibition of MKK6 by the clinically important MKK1/2 inhibitor trametinib suggests that even a single off-target may be significant. Depending on the cell type or stimulus, blocking the p38 MAPK pathway may influence survival by promoting oncogenic or tumour suppressive results. Despite the fact that trametinib's IC_{50} for p38 MAPK inhibition was higher than that of MKK1/2-ERK1/2, this concentration range is often used in literature studies. SB203580, a p38 MAPK inhibitor, increased the cell inhibitory response to selumetinib, implying that inhibiting p38 synergizes with MKK1/2 inhibitors to compromise cell viability in melanoma cell lines. CA-MKK6 and p38 MAPK signalling have been shown to shield melanoma cells from UV-induced apoptosis, according to previous research. When SB203580 was combined with trametinib, the synergistic impact was reduced, which we believe is due to trametinib's off-target influence on MKK6. The findings indicate that trametinib's impact on p38 MAPK may enhance the drug's effectiveness in some circumstances.

Finally, they discussed the problem of differential modulation of phosphorylation targets downstream of BRAF-MKK-ERK signalling. Different proteomics studies sometimes see differences in phosphosite responses to the same pathway, but cannot differentiate if such results are due to unequal signalling responses or experimental heterogeneity. The findings revealed that various cell systems had different reactions to the same pathway. However, some of the reported inconsistencies may be explained by methodological differences between laboratories or off-target inhibitor results, which the study could not rule out. The authors were able to re-address this issue more rigorously after comparing four inhibitors using data obtained by one lab in one cell system. Finally, it was discovered that certain, but not all, validated ERK1/2 targets are protected from phosphorylation in cell system. The significance of this discovery is that nothing is known regarding why certain phosphorylation sites that are usually supervised by ERK are bypassed under some conditions but are repeatedly attacked under others. Awareness the processes that regulate variability in cellular responses may include an understanding of the fundamental mechanisms that contribute to differential regulation within the phosphoproteome. The gain of new insight into new targets for control by the oncogenic BRAF driver pathway in cancer cells by comparing different inhibitors of multiple kinase tiers utilising phosphoproteomics, which is a valuable method for assessing the specificity of drugs and drug candidates [50]. The Bender and colleagues have shown that significant effect on CK2 and it has a proliferation and differentiation of neural stem cells from the sub ventricular region in a sample. They reported that proliferative ability is significantly reduced when the enzyme is inhibited [51]. CK2 inhibition interrupts the neuronal and glial lineages within a three-day time window during differentiation. CK2 kinase function seems to be redundant at later levels of differentiation. While it has been established that CK2 plays a role in nervous system production, knowledge on the role of kinase-dependent pathways in neurogenesis is scarce. This may be attributed to the CK2 or CK2 knockout mice's extreme and fatal neurodevelopmental phenotypes. Huillard et al. found that disrupting the CK2 subunit induced oligodendrogenesis to be negatively regulated. The bHLH transcription factor Olig2, which is one of the main regulators of oligodendrocyte growth [52], interacts with CK2. It was also discovered that embryonic stem cells lacking tCK2 had a viability deficiency. They also discovered that CK2 is needed for neurosphere oligodendroglia differentiation. In the absence of CK2, the effect of CK2 is attributed to a defect in the holo enzyme's CK2 kinase activity. Those substrates that are only phosphorylated by the holo enzyme cannot be phosphorylated without CK2. It also explains how Drosophila CK2 is involved in cell proliferation and survival during brain growth. The nucleolar mushroom body miniature (mbm) protein is one of the potential substrates. This protein is thought to be involved in nutrient-dependent signalling processes that regulate ribosomal expression. The observed findings with inhibitors of CK2 kinase activity clearly support the theory that the holo enzyme is the functional type of CK2 involved in neurosphere proliferation and differentiation. Furthermore, hereditary disruption in embryonic neurogenesis results in decreased neural stem cell proliferation and self-renewal. These results are in line with our findings from postnatal neural stem cells originating from the subventricular region that were inhibited. The issue of lethality can be solved by using knock-down methods or CK2 inhibitors, which allows researchers to explore the postnatal function of CK2 in the nervous system. The function of CK2 in the nervous system may be investigated further using these methods. As a result, it was discovered that CK2 plays a role in ion channel organisation and synaptic transmission [51]. CX-4945 [Silmitasertib] is a powerful inhibitor of CK2's kinase function that was developed as an anticancer medication. CX- 4945 has been shown to have cytotoxic properties in acute lymphoblastic leukaemia cells, inhibit pro survival signalling in human breast cancer cells, and may be used to treat cancer stem cells in glioblastomas. CX-4945 also appears to control osteoblast differentiation *in vitro* and can function as a splicing regulator. CX-4945-treated human mesenchymal stem cells divide into adipocytes in the same way as untreated cells do, according to a new report. The inability to prevent differentiation was shown to be followed by a lack of CK2 kinase inhibitory activity. The function of CK2 in neurogenesis was investigated using CX-4945 in various concentrations. The proliferation of neurospheres is inhibited in a dose-dependent way, according to this research. Since CK2 can be effectively inhibited, two concentrations, 10 and 20 M, were chosen for differentiation experiments. A higher concentration of CX 4945 causes apoptosis, which greatly decreases cell numbers and attacks stem cells and neuronal precursor cells in particular.

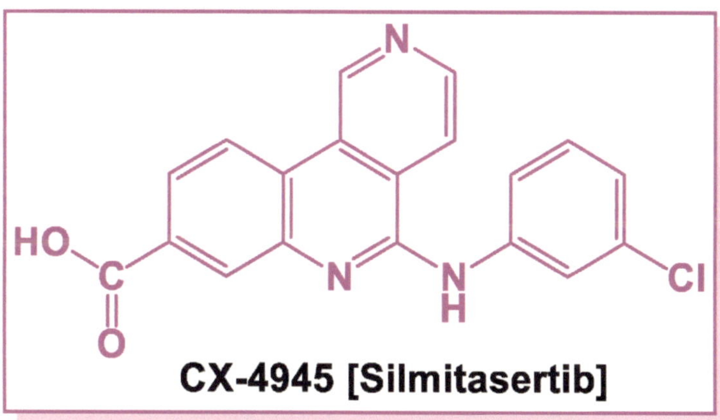

As a result, the effect on neurogenesis at this concentration is due to apoptosis rather than a particular inhibition. Despite this, the remaining cells maintain their cell cycle distribution. We were able to demonstrate that inhibiting CK2 contributes to a significant suppression of neurogenesis as well as a reduction in gliogenesis by focusing on the surviving cells during differentiation. We have also seen that the effect of CK2 persists for many days during separation and that this effect degrades slowly and steadily. The lack of apoptosis was observed when a dosage of 10 M CX-4945 was used, indicating that this concentration is non-toxic. In this scenario, we found that gliogenesis was inhibited but not neurogenesis, indicating that neuronal precursors are more susceptible to apoptosis at higher inhibitor concentrations. Using various concentrations of quinalizarin, they were able to achieve either heavy apoptosis or no inhibition of the CK2 kinase activity. The CK2 kinase function was inhibited by about 40% when 40 M quinalizarin was used. In this event, neurogenesis was inhibited but gliogenesis was not. The findings obtained with the two inhibitors lead me to believe that neurogenesis inhibition is somehow linked to apoptosis activation, whereas gliogenesis inhibition is specifically linked to CK2 inhibition. This hypothesis is confirmed by Huillard and Ziercher's findings, which showed that disrupting CK2 subunit expression causes oligo-dendrogenesis to be negatively controlled. It appears that the period when CK2 kinase activity is needed for differentiation is critical. Although knocking out CK2 in embryonic stem cells causes overall developmental failure, lineage finding can benefit from timely activation or inhibition of the enzyme within a particular organ system, particularly when the enzyme is partially up- or down-regulated. The results indicate that inhibiting CK2 for 1–3 days prevents stem cell differentiation. The interdependencies of the specific partners, such as neurons and glial cells, are also a significant feature of CK2's function in neurogenesis. Glial cells are well known for producing a wide variety of trophic factors and cytokines that can aid in the survival and differentiation of neurons. The current observations in the nervous system are consistent with the osteoclast separation results obtained with CX-4945. Furthermore, CX-4945 was found to suppress RANKL-induced osteoblast differentiation. CX-4945, on the other hand, increased BMP2-induced osteoblast differentiation. Another research looked at the differentiation of pre-adipocytes into adipocytes and found that the activation of the CK2 kinase increased at the start of the differentiation phase and decreased as the differentiation progressed. Furthermore, inhibiting CK2 kinase activity at the start of differentiation for up to 6 days inhibits differentiation, although there was no inhibition of differentiation after day 6. As a consequence, these findings are in strong harmony with the neural differentiation evidence discussed here. Future experiments with graded up- and down-regulations of CK2 will reveal whether CK2 is still active in the differentiation fate decision of neurons and glial cells [51].

Platelet glycoprotein IIb/IIIa inhibitors (GP IIb/IIIa inhibitors) have a well-established thrombolytic role in myocardial infarction. Despite this, there is a scarcity of information on the mechanism of GP IIb/IIIa inhibitors'cardioprotective function in ischemic-reperfusion injury (IR). 120 minutes of coronary ischemia and 180 minutes of reperfusion were provided to Sprague–Dawley rats. PKC (chelerythrine), PI3 kinase and Akt (wortmannin), p38 MAPK (SB203582), p42/44 MAPK (PD98059), and ERK1/2 (u0126) inhibitors were provided by continuous intravenous infusion at a rate of 2 ug/kg/min 30 minutes prior to reperfusion with/without inhibitors of PKC (chelerythrine), PI3 kinase and Western blot analysis was used to isolate and analyse proteins. The apoptotic index (AI) was determined as the percentage of myocytes positive for terminal deoxynucleotidyltransferase-mediated dUTP-biotin nick-end labelling of all myocytes stained with 4′, 6-diamidino-2-phenylindole and the ratio of myocardial necrotic region to the area at risk (AAR). The GP IIb/IIIa inhibitor decreased the ratio of myocardial necrotic region to AAR and AI, as well as exerting an immediate cardioprotective impact by phosphorylating and triggering multiple signalling pathways such as PKC, PI3 kinase, Akt, p38 MAPK, p42/44 MAPK, and ERK1/2. Raf and MEK1/2 phosphorylation, on the other hand, did not show any major rises. Chang et al., found that inhibiting GP IIb/IIIa decreased the level of cardiac IR and greatly reduced myocyte apoptosis in rats. Furthermore, the cardioprotective influence was induced by several signal transduction pathways activation [53].

Linagliptin-induced vasodilation was studied by Seo et al., in a concentration-dependent manner. The absence of endothelium, as well as pre-treatment with a nitric oxide synthase inhibitor (L-NAME) or a small-conductance Ca^{2+}-activated K^+ channel inhibitor, had little impact on the vasodilatory effect of linagliptin (apamin). Furthermore, the adenylyl cyclase inhibitor SQ22536, the protein kinase A (PKA) inhibitor KT5720, the guanylylcyclase inhibitor ODQ, and the protein kinase G (PKG) inhibitor KT5823 had no impact on linagliptin's vasodilatory effect. Y-27632, on the other hand, greatly reduced linagliptin-induced vasodilation by inhibiting Rho-associated protein kinase. The function of ion channels in linagliptin's vasodilatory effect was also examined. Glibenclamide (ATP-sensitive K^+ channels), Ba^{2+} (inwardly rectifying K^+ channels), 4-AP (voltage-dependent K^+ channels), and paxilline (large conductance Ca^{2+}-activated K^+ channels) were not found to influence linagliptin-induced vasodilation. Furthermore, nifedipine, an inhibitor of L-type Ca^{2+} channels, and thapsigargin, an inhibitor of the sarcoplasmic/endoplasmic reticulum Ca^{2+}-ATPase (SERCA) pump, had no impact on linagliptin's vasodilatory effect. The inhibition of Rho-associated kinase, but not the endothelium, cAMP-PKA or cGMP-PKG-dependent signalling pathways, K^+ channels, Ca^{2+} influx, or the SERCA pump, could be responsible for linagliptin-induced vasodilation [54].

PKCs are thought to control certain pancreatic functions in natural acinar cells, ductal cells, and islets, as well as in disease states such as insulin tolerance, diabetes mellitus, pancreatitis, and pancreatic ductal adenocarcinoma, according to Fleming and Storz (PDA). PKCs control secretory processes in the regular pancreas, as shown by amylase secretion in acinar cells, bicarbonate secretion in ductal cells, and glucagon and insulin secretion in islets. PKCs play a role in the production of insulin tolerance and diabetes mellitus by regulating -cell proliferation and activity, as well as insulin secretion and cell death. PKCs play a crucial role in pancreatic injury and inflammation, as well as trypsinogen activation and basolateral exocytosis, during pancreatitis. PKCs eventually play a role in the growth of PDA by promoting acinar cell dedifferentiation (PKC) and acinar-to-ductal metaplasia (PKC). PKC control proliferation and promote anchorage-independent development throughout the progression of PDA. Atypical PKCs have also been linked to the regulation of metastasis. In conclusion, PKC isoforms play a variety of roles in normal pancreatic regulation, but they may also play a role in the onset and development of pancreatic disease [55].

Mitochondrial ATP synthase, a significant ATP supply in respiring cells, should be regulated in both quantity and action to react to differing ATP demands. Sugawara et al., screened 80 protein kinase inhibitors and discovered that four of them decreased mitochondrial ATP synthesis function in HeLa cells. Knocking down their target kinases (PKA, PKCd, CaMKII, and smMLCK) consistently resulted in lower mitochondrial ATP synthesis output. The mitochondria of smMLCK-knockdown cells only possessed a limited amount of ATP synthase, whereas the a- and b-subunits of ATP synthase were formed normally, implying that smMLCK affects ATP synthase assembly (or decay) [56].

PIM (proviral insertion in murine) Kinases are a kind of proto-oncogene that phosphorylates the target proteins' serine/threonine residues. PIM-1, PIM-2, and PIM-3 are the three groups that play an important regulatory function in signal transduction cascades by facilitating cell survival, proliferation, and drug tolerance. These kinases are overexpressed in a variety of solid and hematopoietic tumours, supporting malignant cell growth and survival *in vitro* and *in vivo* by controlling cell cycle and inhibiting apoptosis. They are constitutively active until transcribed and they lack a regulatory domain. PIM kinases are thought to be essential downstream effectors of oncoproteins that overexpress and aid in the mediation of drug resistance to available agents like rapamycin. According to Panchal and Sabina, PIM kinases have special hinge regions where two Prolines exist, which makes ATP binding unique while also providing a focus for a growing array of potent PIM kinase inhibitors. Preclinical trials of such inhibitory compounds in different cancers suggest that they have positive efficacy, and some of them are currently being studied. In their study, they described the molecular mechanism and signalling mechanisms of PIM kinases, as well as matriculation in multiple cancers and a list of commonly used inhibitors [57]. Dengue virus (DENV) infection is a disease that is common to many areas of the world, and its rising incidence places it among the diseases that pose a serious public health danger. Dengue fever (DF), dengue hemorrhagic fever (DHF), and dengue shock syndrome are among the clinical symptoms of DENV infection (DSS). Extreme dengue fever is characterised by increased proinflammatory cytokines and vascular permeability, all of which trigger organ damage. Sreekanth et al. used hepatic cell lines, mouse models, and autopsy specimens from DENV-infected patients to observe symptoms of liver damage, and these signs substantiated the results of inflammatory responses and hepatic cell apoptosis. During viral infections, MAPK are implicated in inflammatory responses and cellular tension. MAPK signalling has been implicated in inflammatory responses and hepatic cell apoptosis in both *in vitro* and *in vivo* models, according to published evidence. In DENV infection, modifying MAPK signalling reduces inflammatory responses and hepatic cell apoptosis. This body of knowledge about the function of MAPK signalling in inflammatory responses and cell apoptosis in DENV infection is illuminating, and it could speed up the creation of new or repositioned therapies to treat this unpredictably disabling disorder [58].

11. Conclusion

In this study, we have addressed the role of protein kinase in human cells and the effects of protein kinase inhibitors in the treatment of various diseases and disorders. Protein kinase is a type of kinase enzyme that adds phosphate groups to other proteins chemically (i.e. phosphorylation). Many biochemical signalling pathways within cells (i.e. signal transduction) and effectors in cellular functions, such as cell proliferation and necrosis, are influenced by this enzyme. Protein kinases are the third messenger mechanism, and most of their isoforms depend on second messengers like cAMP and calcium to function. Overexpression of protein kinase, on the other hand, causes life-threatening diseases such as cancer, cardiovascular disease (hypertension), central nervous system disease, skin disease (inflammation), diabetes mellitus, and so on. Moreover, the findings of various researchers has also added to the fact. There are currently a range of protein kinase inhibitors in the market that inhibit protein kinase activity. They can be used to regulate the cellular responses that protein kinase activity causes. As a result, there is scope for the design and production of new medicines that inhibit protein kinase overexpression for the prevention and treatment of associated disorders. The functions of protein kinases in signal transduction, the effects of overexpression, and the therapeutic roles of various protein kinase inhibitors are all discussed here. As a result, further research into the protein kinase is needed in order to develop more potent and effective prophylactics for disease treatment.

Abbreviations

ATP	Adenosinetriphosphate
ADP	Adenosinediphosphate
PTMs	Post-transitional modifications
JAK	Januskinase
MAPK	Mitogen-activated protein kinase
CDKs	Cyclin-dependent kinases
Abl	Abelsonmurine leukaemia virus
MKK4	Mitogen-activatedproteinkinase4
AMPK	AMP-activated protein kinase

VEGFR	Vascular endothelial growth factor receptors
EGFR	Epidermal growth factor receptors
NAFLD/NASH	Non-alcoholic fatty liver disease/Non-alcoholic steatohepatitis
LRRK2	Leucine-richrepeatkinase2
NO	Nitricoxide
PKI	protein kinase inhibitor
ALI	Acute lung inflammation acute lung inflammation
ERK	Extracellular signal related kinase
PD	Parkinson's disease

Author details

Panneerselvam Theivendren[1*], Selvaraj Kunjiappan[2], Yashoda Mariappa Hegde[3], Sivakumar Vellaichamy[4], Muruganathan Gopal[5], Senthil Rajan Dhramalingam[3] and Sattanathan Kumar[1]

1 Department of Pharmaceutical Chemistry, Swamy Vivekananda College of Pharmacy, Namakkal, Tamilnadu, India

2 Department of Biotechnology, Kalasalingam Academy of Research and Education, Krishnankoil, India

3 Department of Pharmaceutics, Swamy Vivekananda College of Pharmacy, Namakkal, Tamilnadu, India

4 Department of Pharmaceutics, Arulmigu Kalasalingam College of Pharmacy, Krishnankoil, India

5 Department of Pharmacognosy, Swamy Vivekananda College of Pharmacy, Namakkal, Tamilnadu, India

*Address all correspondence to: tpsphc@gmail.com

References

[1] Manning G, Whyte DB, Martinez R, Hunter T, Sudarsanam S. The protein kinase complement of the human genome. Science 2002;298:1912-34.

[2] Ubersax JA, Ferrell Jr JE. Mechanisms of specificity in protein phosphorylation. Nature reviews Molecular cell biology 2007;8:530-41.

[3] Manning G, Whyte D, Martinez R, Hunter T, Sudarsanam S. cAMP-dependent protein kinase from Plasmodium falciparum: an update. Trends in Biochemical Sciences 2002;27:514-20.

[4] Alberts B. Molecular biology of the cell. Garland science; 2008.

[5] Krebs EG. The phosphorylation of proteins: a major mechanism for biological regulation. Biochem Soc Trans 1985;13:813-20.

[6] Turk BE. Understanding and exploiting substrate recognition by protein kinases. Current opinion in chemical biology 2008;12:4-10.

[7] Patterson H, Nibbs R, McInnes I, Siebert S. Protein kinase inhibitors in the treatment of inflammatory and autoimmune diseases. Clinical & Experimental Immunology 2014;176:1-10.

[8] Burke JE. Structural basis for regulation of phosphoinositide kinases and their involvement in human disease. Molecular cell 2018;71:653-73.

[9] Sun R, Wang L. Thymidine kinase 2 enzyme kinetics elucidate the mechanism of thymidine-induced mitochondrial DNA depletion. Biochemistry 2014;53:6142-50.

[10] Roskoski Jr R. ERK1/2 MAP kinases: structure, function, and regulation. Pharmacological research 2012;66:105-43.

[11] Schwartz PA, Murray BW. Protein kinase biochemistry and drug discovery. Bioorganic chemistry 2011;39:192-210.

[12] Nishi H, Shaytan A, Panchenko AR. Physicochemical mechanisms of protein regulation by phosphorylation. Frontiers in genetics 2014;5:270.

[13] Kathryn LM. Pathophysiology: The Biologic Basis for Disease in Adults and Children, 7e: Elsevier, Mosby; 2014.

[14] Heinrich R, Neel BG, Rapoport TA. Mathematical models of protein kinase signal transduction. Molecular cell 2002;9:957-70.

[15] Miller ML, Jensen LJ, Diella F, Jørgensen C, Tinti M, Li L, et al. Linear motif atlas for phosphorylation-dependent signaling. Science signaling 2008;1:ra2-ra.

[16] Hunter T. Tyrosine phosphorylation: thirty years and counting. Current opinion in cell biology 2009;21:140-6.

[17] Capra M, Nuciforo PG, Confalonieri S, Quarto M, Bianchi M, Nebuloni M, et al. Frequent alterations in the expression of serine/threonine kinases in human cancers. Cancer research 2006;66:8147-54.

[18] Dhanasekaran N, Reddy EP. Signaling by dual specificity kinases. Oncogene 1998;17:1447-55.

[19] Jin J, Pawson T. Modular evolution of phosphorylation-based signalling systems. Philosophical Transactions of the Royal Society B: Biological Sciences 2012;367:2540-55.

[20] Pearce LR, Komander D, Alessi DR. The nuts and bolts of AGC protein kinases. Nature reviews Molecular cell biology 2010;11:9-22.

[21] Wayman GA, Tokumitsu H, Davare MA, Soderling TR. Analysis of

CaM-kinase signaling in cells. Cell calcium 2011;50:1-8.

[22] Eide EJ, Virshup DM. Casein kinase I: another cog in the circadian clockworks. Chronobiology international 2001;18:389-98.

[23] Cohen P, Goedert M. GSK3 inhibitors: development and therapeutic potential. Nature reviews Drug discovery 2004;3:479-87.

[24] Moeslein FM, Myers MP, Landreth GE. The CLK family kinases, CLK1 and CLK2, phosphorylate and activate the tyrosine phosphatase, PTP-1B. Journal of Biological Chemistry 1999;274:26697-704.

[25] Müller-Taubenberger A, Ishikawa-Ankerhold HC, Kastner PM, Burghardt E, Gerisch G. The STE group kinase SepA controls cleavage furrow formation in Dictyostelium. Cell motility and the cytoskeleton 2009;66:929-39.

[26] Abdi AI, Carvalho TG, Wilkes JM, Doerig C. A secreted Plasmodium falciparum kinase reveals a signature motif for classification of tyrosine kinase-like kinases. Microbiology 2013;159:2533-47.

[27] Pal A, Pal A, Mallick AI, Biswas P, Chatterjee P. Molecular characterization of Bu-1 and TLR2 gene in Haringhata Black chicken. Genomics 2020;112:472-83.

[28] Hornberg JJ, Bruggeman FJ, Binder B, Geest CR, De Vaate AMB, Lankelma J, et al. Principles behind the multifarious control of signal transduction: ERK phosphorylation and kinase/phosphatase control. The FEBS journal 2005;272:244-58.

[29] Jia C, Bai J, Liu Z, Gao S, Han Y, Yan H. Application of a titanium-based metal-organic framework to protein kinase activity detection and inhibitor screening. Analytica Chimica Acta 2020;1128:99-106.

[30] Steinberg SF. Post-translational modifications at the ATP-positioning G-loop that regulate protein kinase activity. Pharmacological research 2018;135:181-7.

[31] Klövekorn P, Pfaffenrot B, Juchum M, Selig R, Albrecht W, Zender L, et al. From off-to on-target: New BRAF-inhibitor-template-derived compounds selectively targeting mitogen activated protein kinase kinase 4 (MKK4). European Journal of Medicinal Chemistry 2021;210:112963.

[32] Qiao Y, Chen T, Yang H, Chen Y, Lin H, Qu W, et al. Small molecule modulators targeting protein kinase CK1 and CK2. European journal of medicinal chemistry 2019;181: 111581.

[33] Ding R, Wu W, Sun Z, Li Z. AMP-activated protein kinase: An attractive therapeutic target for ischemia-reperfusion injury. European Journal of Pharmacology 2020:173484.

[34] Roskoski Jr R. Properties of FDA-approved small molecule protein kinase inhibitors: A 2020 update. Pharmacological research 2020;152:104609.

[35] Gaji RY, Sharp AK, Brown AM. Protein kinases in Toxoplasma gondii. International Journal for Parasitology 2021.

[36] Zhao P, Saltiel AR. From overnutrition to liver injury: AMP-activated protein kinase in nonalcoholic fatty liver diseases. Journal of Biological Chemistry 2020;295:12279-89.

[37] Alghamdi F, Alshuweishi Y, Salt IP. Regulation of nutrient uptake by AMP-activated protein kinase. Cellular Signalling 2020:109807.

[38] Li X, Liu R, Zhang L, Jiang Z. The emerging role of AMP-activated protein kinase in cholestatic liver diseases. Pharmacological research 2017;125:105-13.

[39] Lee S-H, Suk K. Emerging roles of protein kinases in microglia-mediated neuroinflammation. Biochemical pharmacology 2017;146:1-9.

[40] Diering S, Stathopoulou K, Goetz M, Rathjens L, Harder S, Piasecki A, et al. Receptor-independent modulation of cAMP-dependent protein kinase and protein phosphatase signaling in cardiac myocytes by oxidizing agents. Journal of Biological Chemistry 2020;295:15342-65.

[41] Ghione S, Mabrouk N, Paul C, Bettaieb A, Plenchette S. Protein kinase inhibitor-based cancer therapies: Considering the potential of nitric oxide (NO) to improve cancer treatment. Biochemical pharmacology 2020;176:113855.

[42] Mori A, Ishikawa E, Amano T, Sakamoto K, Nakahara T. Anti-diabetic drug metformin dilates retinal blood vessels through activation of AMP-activated protein kinase in rats. European journal of pharmacology 2017;798:66-71.

[43] Yılmaz S. P. 762 KN-93, an inhibitor of ca++/calmodulin-dependent protein kinase, inhibits neuronal cell viability in an in vitro Alzheimer's disease model. European Neuropsychopharmacology 2020;40:S431-S2.

[44] Abedi F, Hayes AW, Reiter R, Karimi G. Acute lung injury: The therapeutic role of Rho kinase inhibitors. Pharmacological research 2020;155:104736.

[45] Ahmed T, Zulfiqar A, Arguelles S, Rasekhian M, Nabavi SF, Silva AS, et al. Map kinase signaling as therapeutic target for neurodegeneration. Pharmacological research 2020:105090.

[46] Gordon R, Singh N, Lawana V, Ghosh A, Harischandra DS, Jin H, et al. Protein kinase Cδ upregulation in microglia drives neuroinflammatory responses and dopaminergic neurodegeneration in experimental models of Parkinson's disease. Neurobiology of disease 2016;93:96-114.

[47] Lund S, Porzgen P, Mortensen AL, Hasseldam H, Bozyczko-Coyne D, Morath S, et al. Inhibition of microglial inflammation by the MLK inhibitor CEP-1347. Journal of neurochemistry 2005;92:1439-51.

[48] Wu C, Watts ME, Rubin LL. MAP4K4 activation mediates motor neuron degeneration in amyotrophic lateral sclerosis. Cell reports 2019;26:1143-56. e5.

[49] Watts ME, Wu C, Rubin LL. Suppression of MAP4K4 signaling ameliorates motor neuron degeneration in amyotrophic lateral sclerosis-molecular studies toward new therapeutics. Journal of experimental neuroscience 2019;13:11790695 19862798.

[50] Basken J, Stuart SA, Kavran AJ, Lee T, Ebmeier CC, Old WM, et al. Specificity of phosphorylation responses to mitogen activated protein (MAP) kinase pathway inhibitors in melanoma cells. Molecular & Cellular Proteomics 2018;17:550-64.

[51] Bender M, Schwind L, Grundmann D, Martin M, Klotz M, Götz C, et al. Impact of protein kinase CK2 inhibitors on proliferation and differentiation of neural stem cells. Heliyon 2017;3:e00318.

[52] Wang X, Gupta P, Fairbanks J, Hansen D. Protein kinase CK2 both promotes robust proliferation and inhibits the proliferative fate in the C. elegans germ line. Developmental biology 2014;392:26-41.

[53] Barlow K, Thomson E, Johnson D, Minns R, Carter J, Mungala Odera V, et al. Critical care outcomes. Current Opinion in Critical Care 2006;12:489-526.

[54] Seo MS, Li H, An JR, Jang JH, Jung HS, Kim T, et al. The vasodilatory effect of the antidiabetic drug linagliptin via inhibition of Rho-associated protein kinase in aortic smooth muscle. Life sciences 2019;219:1-10.

[55] Fleming AK, Storz P. Protein kinase C isoforms in the normal pancreas and in pancreatic disease. Cellular signalling 2017;40:1-9.

[56] Sugawara K, Fujikawa M, Yoshida M. Screening of protein kinase inhibitors and knockdown experiments identified four kinases that affect mitochondrial ATP synthesis activity. FEBS letters 2013;587:3843-7.

[57] Panchal NK, Sabina E. A serine/threonine protein PIM kinase as a biomarker of cancer and a target for anticancer therapy. Life Sciences 2020:117866.

[58] Ojha CR, Rodriguez M, Karuppan MKM, Lapierre J, Kashanchi F, El-Hage N. Toll-like receptor 3 regulates Zika virus infection and associated host inflammatory response in primary human astrocytes. PLoS One 2019;14:e0208543.

Chapter 6

Recent Advances in the Therapeutic Development of Receptor Tyrosine Kinases (RTK) against Different Types of Cancer

Somi Patranabis

Abstract

Receptor Tyrosine Kinases (RTKs) are an important class of receptors involved in regulating different cellular functions. The usual pathway of RTK activation involves specific ligand binding, dimerization and trans-autophosphorylation. Recently, RTK has been extensively studied as they have potential applications in targeted cancer therapy. RTK-based therapeutic strategies are promising because dysfunction of RTK is connected to a variety of diseases. More specifically, RTK has been widely associated with different types of cancer and related diseases. The chapter aims to cover recent advances and challenges in RTK related research, to get an overview of the problems and possibilities associated with targeted therapy. This will help in deciphering novel therapeutic applications in the future.

Keywords: receptor tyrosine kinase, RTK mutations, cancer, targeted therapy, RTK inhibitors

1. Introduction

A cell is dependent on a wide array of molecules to perform all its activities in a regulated manner. Any disruption in any of the molecules or related pathways can lead to various developmental issues and diseases. Hence, a cell depends on stringent signaling pathways which enables it to grow, proliferate, differentiate, and carry out all physiological processes required for survival and/or apoptosis. One such signaling pathway is the Receptor Tyrosine Kinase (RTK) signaling pathway which is extremely crucial in almost all kind of cells. This pathway usually begins by activation of receptors on the cell membrane, which in turn, undergoes self-phosphorylation and activation of other downstream signaling targets (**Figure 1**). There are various mechanisms by which RTK can elicit its effects on the cell. Any mutation in RTK or its associated targets can be detrimental to the cell, leading to various diseases, including cancer. Thus, identifying these mutations and strategizing therapies targeting such receptors and their associated molecules, can prove to pave the path for creating effective anticancer drugs. Tyrosine kinase inhibitors can also be used to attenuate the increased activity of RTK signaling pathway. A multitude of cancers have been linked to dysregulation of RTK signaling. This chapter covers the current scenario of RTK-associated cancers and the recent therapeutic

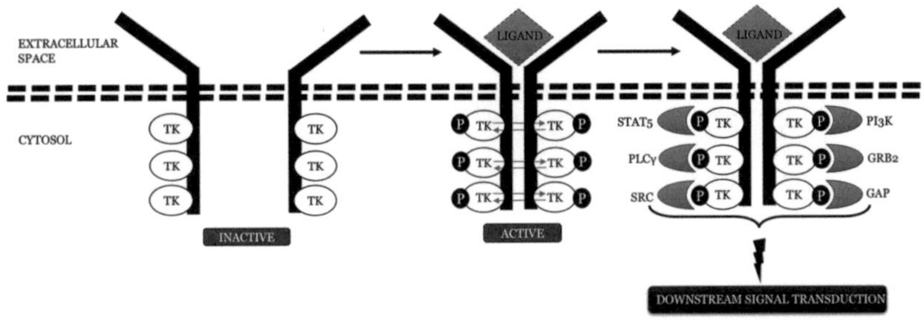

Figure 1.
Mechanism of activation of the tyrosine kinase receptor. Receptor tyrosine kinase exists as monomers in the inactive state. It has an extracellular domain and a cytosolic domain. Upon binding to a specific ligand, it is activated by trans-autophosphorylation of the tyrosine kinase domain. This leads to recruitment of specific adaptor protein(s) and activation of downstream signaling pathways.

strategies, either implemented or having the capacity to be implemented in the future. An understanding of the recent advances in this field has ample potential to investigate the plethora of possibilities ahead.

2. RTK: at the crossroads of cell growth, proliferation and differentiation

Receptor Tyrosine Kinases are a class of very important receptors involved in signaling mechanisms related to cell growth, proliferation, survival and development. Dysregulation of this receptor or its associated molecules has been linked to various diseases, including cancer. Human genome contains around 55 receptor tyrosine kinases (RTK). These RTKs undergo several types of post-translational modifications, some of which include tyrosine phosphorylation, ubiquitination, ectodomain shedding, and regulated intramembrane proteolysis. Structurally RTKs are single-pass membrane proteins that are grouped into subfamilies based on similarity in their extracellular domains. The intracellular kinase domains are in turn, coupled to different extracellular modules. Many RTKs have been reported to be cleaved by gamma-secretase-mediated intramembrane proteolysis. It is a two-step process. In the first step, the RTK ectodomain is released to the extracellular space by proteolytic cleavage called shedding. In the second step, RTK transmembrane domain is cleaved by the gamma-secretase complex. This, in turn, leads to release of a soluble RTK intracellular domain that can translocate to various cellular compartments, such as the nucleus or proteasome, and can also interact with transcriptional regulators and other molecules to induce cell survival, proliferation and differentiation. The tyrosine kinase domain is an integral part of this intracellular domain [1]. The internalization process retains the RTK's transmembrane domain. The endosomal RTK remains active before being recycled or degraded. The transport of RTK from endosome-Golgi-ER to the nucleus is primarily dependent on membranous vesicles and hence, relies on its interaction with the transport complexes like COP-I vesicle complex, Sec61 translocon complex and importin. Nuclear- RTKs have the property of retaining oncogenic properties and can enhance cancer progression. Nuclear-localized RTKs have, in fact, positive correlation with cancer recurrence and therapeutic resistance of cancer patients [2]. It has also been observed that reduced ectodomain shedding and decreased ubiquitination of the cytoplasmic region produce malignant cells. Events like receptor phosphorylation and ubiquitination are reversible, whereas proteolytic cleavage events are irreversible. Any such modification has the potential to alter the subcellular localization of RTKs [3].

The activation of RTK is by dimerization of two monomers and this can either be receptor-mediated or ligand-mediated. The ligands can either be soluble or membrane-embedded. Sometimes, multiple ligands can interact with the same receptor. Such ligands often act as biased agonists and can initiate signaling responses via activation of the same receptor [4]. Activation of RTK involves homodimerization followed by trans autophosphorylation. However, some groups of RTKs can interact with each other even in the absence of ligand, which eventually leads to heterodimerization across sub-families. This results in irreproducibility of data from different experimental sets and hence, is a big hurdle for RTK inhibitors to produce desired therapeutic effects [5]. Both genetic and epigenetic modifications in the genes encoding for RTKs are responsible for activation of growth factor-mediated signaling events. This hyperactivation of RTK mediated signaling cascades can even cause cancer [6].

The degree and duration of RTK signaling plays a pivotal role in determining specific cellular behaviors. The feedback regulation of RTK signaling is critical for determining different diseases. The loss of such feedback mechanism can lead to an aberrant increase in the RTK signaling, resulting in an uncontrolled increase in cell growth, proliferation and survival. Thus, both positive and negative regulators of RTK signaling are crucial in development [7].

The use of Tyrosine Kinase Inhibitors (TKI) remains one of the standard methods of elucidating anticancer effects. The antitumoral properties of TKIs due to induction of apoptosis and cell cycle arrest is a result of tightly controlled events involving different cellular compartments such as endoplasmic reticulum and mitochondria [8].

3. RTK mutations: targets for cancer therapy

Receptor Tyrosine Kinase and its downstream signaling mechanism is crucial for maintaining the integrity of cellular processes, such as growth, proliferation and survival. Any mutation in the RTK or its associated partners can be detrimental to the cell and can even be oncogenic in nature. A mutation which can directly or indirectly lead to upregulation of RTK can eventually result in tumor formation. Recent large-scale genomic studies have highlighted the presence of mutations and alterations in the genes encoding RTKs such as EGFR, HER2/ErbB2, and MET and many other genes. Abnormal RTK activation in human cancers can occur by four major pathways: gain-of-function mutations, genomic amplification, chromosomal rearrangements, and/or autocrine activation [9].

For instance, loss or inactivation of phosphate and tensin homolog (PTEN), leads to overactivation of RTK/PI3K/Akt signaling pathway, eventually leading to tumorigenesis. It has been observed that transcription of PTEN pseudogene, PTENP1, results in sense and antisense transcripts which can, in turn, exhibit post-transcriptional and transcriptional modulation of PTEN expression, respectively. Thus, the effects of the sense and antisense transcripts of PTENP1 on PTEN expression can influence RTK expression and associated signaling pathway, and has promising potential in cancer therapeutics [10]. Another well studied mutant of RTK is MET, which was discovered way back in 1984. The MET RTK and its ligand HGF are key players in more than one type of cancer. High expression of the MET receptor has been shown to correlate with poor prognosis and resistance to therapy. MET exon 14 splicing variants that was initially identified in lung cancer can be treated through various tyrosine kinase inhibitors (TKIs) [11].

Additionally, alternative splicing of RTK pre-mRNA is a novel aspect of study, which can be linked to development of tumor and its maintenance. However, the exact biological functions of different RTK splice variants and the signals responsible for it is not yet well studied. The mechanism by which these splicing events affect the response of tumor to RTK targeted therapies, and whether these therapies have any effect on the fate of RTK alternative splicing, is a very interesting aspect that can be studied. Moreover, the upstream signals that control their expression in tumors, remain to be understood. More importantly, it remains to be determined whether, and how, these splicing events may affect the response of tumor cells to RTK-targeted therapies, and inversely, whether these therapies may impact these splicing events [12].

An overall understanding of the different mutations and alterations related to RTK, will provide a deeper understanding of the receptor and pathways that have important implications in anticancer therapies. Numerous RTK-targeted therapies have been developed to counteract this hyperactivation.

4. RTK disruption in different types of cancer

Receptor Tyrosine kinases are a class of extremely important receptors, and hence, any issue with its regulation or expression can bring about changes in a cell's growth, survival, differentiation and metabolism. One of the most significant effects of RTK dysregulation is cancer and related phenotypes. RTKs serve as important biomarkers that can help analyze tumor progression and metastasis and determine diagnosis and prognosis in the patients. Different cancers have been observed to have a major link with RTKs. For instance, the Epidermal Growth Factor receptor (EGFR) gene has a tyrosine kinase domain, and somatic mutations within this domain, has been linked to non-small cell lung cancer (NSCLC) progression and are called "EGFR sensitizing mutations". One of its inhibitors, called Raf Kinase Inhibitor Protein (RKIP) has the potential to modulate RTK associated signaling events, such as those controlled by EGFR. It has been reported to have metastasis suppressor role in lung cancer [13].

RTK has also been studied extensively in a complex and heterogenous tumor arising from neural crest derived peripheral neurons, known as neuroblastoma, which sadly accounts for 10–15% of all childhood related cancer deaths. Neuroblastoma tumorigenesis involves a receptor tyrosine kinase known as Anaplastic Lymphoma Kinase (ALK), which is a fusion partner in translocation events related to different types of cancers. RTK translocations are responsible for creating a fusion protein containing a dimerizing partner fused to an RTK kinase domain. This, in turn, leads to constitutive kinase domain activation and results in altered RTK cellular localization as well as upregulation of different downstream signaling. In neuroblastoma, however, the full length ALK RTK is itself mutated [14]. Fortunately, many different RTK inhibitors, that are known to inhibit ALK, have been FDA approved and can be used in ALK-driven neuroblastoma treatment.

Apart from neuroblastoma, another type of cancer-related to the brain is gliomas, representing the most common form of malignant brain tumor. Unregulated RTKs such as MET and EGFR, have a central role in the progression of glioblastoma. Mutations in MET and its various regulatory molecules have been linked to different stages of glioblastoma. MET along with its ligand Hepatocyte Growth Factor (HGF) have been shown to hold importance in proliferation, invasion, migration, angiogenesis, recurrence and therapeutic resistance. Targeting HGF/MET in glioma patients is an important therapeutic strategy [15]. HGF/MET has also been extensively studied and found to be involved in different primary malignant brain tumors such as astrocytomas, glioblastomas, oligodendrogliomas, ependymomas, and embryonal central nervous system tumors (including medulloblastomas and others) [16].

Another report highlights the relevance of different types of RTKs such as epidermal growth factor receptor (EGFR), platelet-derived growth factor receptor (PDGFR), c-Met, Tie, Axl, discoidin domain receptor 1 (DDR1), and erythropoietin-producing human hepatocellular carcinoma (Eph) in glioma invasion, and how these can act as targets for glioma therapy [17].

Another common RTK that has been observed in different tumor promoting activities, such as cell proliferation and invasion is AXL. It does so by promoting EMT events, metastasis and drug-resistance. It can also modulate tumor microenvironment and corresponding immune response. This RTK is known to be involved in cancer progression of different types of malignancies ranging from hematopoietic cancers to solid tumors. AXL upregulation has been observed in a wide variety of cancer types, such as breast cancer, and is under focus to investigate possible therapeutic implications by its modulation [18]. Downstream signaling pathways of RTKs such as MAPK, PI3K/Akt and JAK/STAT pathways are major players that regulate cancer progression and metastasis, if not regulated [19]. Problems related to proper regulation of RTK signaling pathway has also been noted in Acute Myeloid Leukemia (AML) [20].

Another type of cancer where issues related to RTK signaling are noted, is osteosarcoma. Multi-target tyrosine kinase inhibitors have shown promising effects in the treatment of osteosarcoma, but the exact target is unclear. This is because inhibiting any one type of RTK as a target for treatment of osteosarcoma has not been proven to be effective. Rather, inhibition of multiple RTKs simultaneously show a much better progress in TKI dependent osteosarcoma treatment. This is because receptor tyrosine kinases like MET, IGF-1R, AXL, PDGFRs, KIT, and FGFRs might be relevant but unimportant targets for osteosarcoma treatment [21].

Gastrointestinal stromal tumor (GIST) is also a type of tumor originating from interstitial cells of Cajal in the GI tract, in which genes encoding RTK are mutated. Genes such as KIT and PDGFRA are activated and eventually lead to tumor formation. It has also been noted that RTK inhibitors like imatinib, can significantly act as therapeutic agent in treatment of patients with GIST [22]. Inhibition of downstream signaling like PI3K/AKT/mTOR also exhibit promising outcomes.

RTK dysregulation has also been observed in head and neck cancers, having important implications in tumorigenesis and metastasis. A recent report illustrates the association of non-coding RNAs with RTK and confirms that RTKs and RTK based therapy are superior to other existing therapeutic interventions for HNC [23].

Although issues in RTK regulation are more common in solid tumors, RTK translocations are also observed in hematological malignancies. Fibroblast Growth Factor Receptor (FGFR), Platelet-Derived Growth Factor Receptor (PDGFR), Rearranged during Transfection (RET), Colony Stimulating Factor 1 Receptor (CSF1R), and Neurotrophic Tyrosine Kinase Receptor Type 3 (NTRK3) fusions are some of the common anomalies found in hematopoietic disorders [24].

5. An overview of RTK inhibitors

There have been a wide variety of Receptor Tyrosine Kinase (RTK) inhibitors, many of which have been approved by the FDA. These inhibitors play a significant role in inhibiting the effect of RTK in cells where they are dysregulated, and thereby, providing a strategy to inhibit cell growth and proliferation. As a result, these inhibitors are well known anticancer agents as well (**Figure 2**). One such example is the inhibitor known as Entrectinib (A) (**Figure 2**), which shows massive

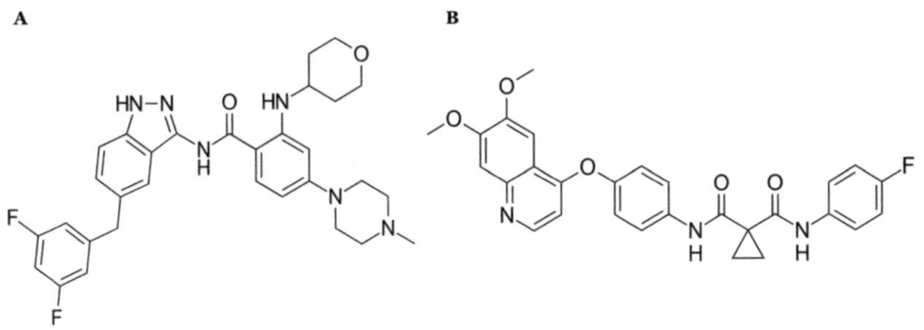

Figure 2.
Structure of potent RTK inhibitors. (A) Entrectinib (B) Cabozantinib.

potential in the treatment of very complex childhood cancer, neuroblastoma. This type of cancer is mainly caused by differential expression of ALK or TRKA/B/C. Entrectinib (RXDX-101) is a pan-ALK, TRKA, TRKB, TRKC, and ROS1 inhibitor with activity against tumors with ALK, NTRK1, NTRK2, NTRK3, and ROS1 alterations in Phase I clinical trials in adults [25]. In June 2019, Entrectinib got its first global approval in Japan, for treating adult and pediatric patients with NTRK fusion-positive and advanced or recurrent solid tumors. It is under regulatory review for the treatment of adult patients with ROS1-positive non-small cell lung cancer (NSCLC). Entrectinib is also under regulatory review in the USA (PDUFA date 18 August 2019) and EU [Priority Medicines (PRIME) designation] for NTRK-positive solid tumors and ROS1-positive NSCLC [26]. Another example of an inhibitor which acts against multiple receptor tyrosine kinases is Cabozantinib (B) (**Figure 2**). This is commercially available as Cabometyx tablet and is used in the treatment of hepatocellular carcinoma (HCC). This inhibitor is usually used in the treatment of patients who are in an advanced stage of cancer and have already been under treatment with the multi-RTK inhibitor sorafenib [27].

6. Promising therapeutic strategies

Receptor Tyrosine Kinases are important regulators of the cell cycle pathway. For a cell to grow and proliferate normally, this receptor plays a major role. Hence, any form of over-expression or overactivity of the RTK or its associated signaling pathway, naturally leads to tumor formation and is well connected with the development of cancer. As a result, RTK and its associated pathways have always been under investigation to find targets in the fight against cancer.

A recent report establishes the relationship between RTK signaling and DNA repair, hinting towards a connection between RTK and the factors involved in the repair pathway. Thus, RTKs can act as potential modulators of the DNA repair pathway and novel therapeutic strategies can be implemented, which will target both DNA repair pathways and RTK mediated signaling pathways [28]. Another report also highlights the link between RTK signaling and DNA repair. Activation of the serine/threonine kinase AKT, also known as protein kinase B (PKB) stimulates DNA repair, like double strand break repair after radiotherapy. Thus, AKT could possibly be a major predictive marker of conventional cancer therapy, molecularly targeted therapy, and immunotherapy for solid tumors. Activated AKT mediates resistance to cancer treatment modalities, such as radiotherapy, chemotherapy, and RTK targeted therapy [29]. Checkpoint inhibitors such as pembrolizumab have proven effective at extending survival for mismatch repair (MMR)-deficient and high microsatellite instability (MSI) metastatic colorectal patients.

Different RTK mutations, deletions, translocations and amplification/overexpressions have been identified and these are currently under study to elucidate their role in cancer. The therapeutic strategies involving RTKs can be classified into small molecule inhibitors and monoclonal antibodies [30].

The presence of RTK fusions is by large, responsible for providing acquired resistance to different therapies. This poses a challenge in the administration of Tyrosine Kinase Inhibitors as anticancer treatment and thus, is a field that requires a lot of attention. Recent reports have come up with the different strategies that can be beneficial in solving this issue [31].

Another interesting and emerging study reveals the connection between EGFR, a common RTK that is dysregulated in different malignancies, and autophagy. In fact, autophagy upregulation as well as downregulation has been observed in several cancers, highlighting its oncogenic and tumor suppressor properties in tumor progression. EGFR has the potential to determine whether autophagy will have a cytotoxic or cytoprotective effect. The EGFR-mediated pathways or proteins involved in autophagy regulation include (a) the EGFR-mTOR pathway; (b) the EGFR-RAS pathway; (c) EGFR-Beclin1; [8] the EGFR-STAT3 pathway and (e) EGFR-LAPTM4B (oncoprotein lysosomal-associated transmembrane protein 4B). Thus, understanding the regulation of autophagy by EGFR can prove to be a highly efficient strategy to identify potential cancer therapeutic targets [32]. Anti-epidermal growth factor receptor (anti-EGFR) agents panitumumab and cetuximab, combined with chemotherapy, have also prolonged the survival of cancer patients.

One of the most promising therapeutic strategy which is widely established and used is immunotherapy. It has proved its worth by improving the prognosis of many patients with a broad variety of hematological and solid malignancies. The importance of immunotherapy has been acknowledged by the Nobel prize for physiology or medicine 2018 awarded for the discovery of cytotoxic T-lymphocyte-associated protein (CTLA-4) to James P. Allison and programmed cell death protein 1/programmed cell death protein ligand 1 (PD-1/PD-L1) to Tasuku Honjo [33].

Epithelial-mesenchymal transition (EMT) is a very important event in the prognosis of malignancy. It has been studied that a receptor tyrosine kinase AXL can directly affect the mesenchymal state, making the tumor more aggressive and drug-resistant. The inhibition of AXL has come up as a promising therapeutic strategy in reversing EMT resensitization to other tyrosine kinase inhibitors, mitotic inhibitors, and platinum-based therapy. Therefore, novel ways to inhibit AXL can be used as an effective therapeutic strategy against different types of cancer [34]. AXL receptor tyrosine kinase (RTK) and its ligand, growth arrest-specific protein 6 (Gas6), have been known to be involved in different malignancies and autoimmune disorders. Several molecules are presently under investigation, which can aid in targeting the AXL/Gas6 molecular system, thus providing therapeutic and diagnostic applications [35].

Apart from the inhibitors that directly target the RTK and its associated molecules, some molecules are naturally present with antitumor properties. One such molecule is decorin, which is present in the tumor microenvironment. This molecule is prototype member of the SLRP family found in a variety of tissues and is expressed in the stroma of various forms of cancer. Decorin has recently gained a lot of attention because of its effects in inflammation, fibrotic disorders, and cancer. Since it is present in the tumor microenvironment, it has been proposed to act as a "guardian from the matrix." Soluble decorin has a pan-RTK inhibiting property and can target a few RTKs, including EGFR, Met, IGF-IR, VEGFR2, and PDGFR. Decorin/RTK interaction can induce caveosomal internalization and receptor degradation. Additionally, this interaction can trigger cell cycle arrest and lead to apoptosis, and can induce conserved catabolic processes, such as endothelial cell autophagy and tumor cell mitophagy. Antimetastatic and antiangiogenic processes have also been reported to be induced by decorin/RTK interaction. Due to such diverse plethora of anticancer effects, decorin is a promising candidate for combatting cancer, especially the cancer types where the major issue is with RTK signaling [36].

Combinations of immunotherapies, RTKs, monoclonal antibodies, and cytotoxic drugs are being investigated to provide broad-spectrum protection against relapse by simultaneously targeting many cancer hallmarks [37].

7. Challenges in RTK related research

Despite the huge potential and success of RTK based targeted cancer therapy, there remain some challenges in this field. One of the major challenges is reducing the off-target effects of Tyrosine Kinase Inhibitors. This non-specificity can lead to deleterious effects on normal cells as well. A possible solution to this challenge can be TKIs-based nanodelivery systems, that will specifically target tumor cells [38]. Another common challenge faced by any anticancer drug is the induction of chemo-resistance during therapy. Patients may invariably develop resistance to these therapies, leading to recurrence. Research that will aim in dealing with chemoresistance by manipulating specific molecules related to it, can have potential role in overcoming this challenge [39]. Thus, increasing target specificity and decreasing drug resistance are the major challenges in RTK related research, along with identification of novel TKIs.

8. Conclusion

This chapter covers the recent advances made in the field of signaling biology, mainly Receptor Tyrosine Kinase-mediated signaling. The structural and functional aspects of the receptor, modes of its activation and current research-based on it has been discussed. Additionally, information related to RTK mutations and disruptions in different types of cancers, gives a better understanding of the different anticancer therapeutic strategies that have come up in the form of inhibitor molecules and drugs. The scope of these receptors is huge if they can be exploited further, along with identification of other novel mutations associated with cancer, and their targets. Sequencing data based on different types of cancer cells, including hematological and solid tumors, can provide a clear picture of the RTK associated genes that are either upregulated or downregulated in different diseases. These studies will open new avenues because different inhibitors/activators or drugs that can target such RTK or its associated molecules, can either be extracted from natural sources or designed in the laboratories. This, in turn, has the potential of targeted therapies and may prove beneficial in the treatment of different types of diseases including cancer.

Author details

Somi Patranabis
Amity Institute of Biotechnology, Amity University, Kolkata, India

*Address all correspondence to: smpatranabis@gmail.com

References

[1] Merilahti J, Elenius K. Gamma-secretase-dependent signaling of receptor tyrosine kinases. Oncogene. 2019 Jan;38(2):151-163.

[2] Chen MK, Hsu JL, Hung MC. Nuclear receptor tyrosine kinase transport and functions in cancer. Adv Cancer Res. 2020;147:59-107.

[3] Kreitman M, Noronha A, Yarden Y. Irreversible modifications of receptor tyrosine kinase. FEBS Lett. 2018 Jul;592(13):2199-2212.

[4] Trenker R, Jura N. Receptor tyrosine kinase activation: From the ligand perspective. Curr Opin Cell Biol. 2020 Apr;63:174-185.

[5] Paul MD, Hristova K. The RTK Interactome: Overview and Perspective on RTK Heterointeractions. Chem Rev. 2019 May 8;119(9):5881-5921.

[6] Spangle JM, Roberts TM. Epigenetic regulation of RTK signaling. J Mol Med (Berl). 2017 Aug;95(8):791-798.

[7] Neben CL, Lo M, Jura N, Klein OD. Feedback regulation of RTK signaling in development. Dev Biol. 2019 Mar 1;447(1):71-89.doi:10.1016/j.ydbio.2017.10.017.

[8] Rodríguez-Hernández MA, de la Cruz-Ojeda P, López-Grueso MJ, Navarro-Villarán E, Requejo-Aguilar R, Castejón-Vega B, Negrete M, Gallego P, Vega-Ochoa Á, Victor VM, Cordero MD, Del Campo JA, Bárcena JA, Padilla CA, Muntané J. Integrated molecular signaling involving mitochondrial dysfunction and alteration of cell metabolism induced by tyrosine kinase inhibitors in cancer. Redox Biol. 2020 Sep;36:101510.

[9] Du Z, Lovly CM. Mechanisms of receptor tyrosine kinase activation in cancer. Mol Cancer. 2018 Feb 19;17(1):58.

[10] Haddadi N, Lin Y, Travis G, Simpson AM, Nassif NT, McGowan EM. PTEN/PTENP1: 'Regulating the regulator of RTK-dependent PI3K/Akt signalling', new targets for cancer therapy. Mol Cancer. 2018 Feb 19;17(1):37.

[11] Malik R, Mambetsariev I, Fricke J, Chawla N, Nam A, Pharaon R, Salgia R. MET receptor in oncology: From biomarker to therapeutic target. Adv Cancer Res. 2020;147:259-301. Adv Cancer Res. 2020;147:259-301.

[12] Whiteside TL. Splice Variants of the RTK Family: Their Role in Tumour Progression and Response to Targeted Therapy. Adv Clin Chem. 2016;74: 103-41.

[13] Raquel-Cunha A, Cardoso-Carneiro D, Reis RM, Martinho O. Current Status of Raf Kinase Inhibitor Protein (RKIP) in Lung Cancer: Behind RTK Signaling. Cells. 2019 May 10;8(5):442.

[14] Umapathy G, Mendoza-Garcia P, Hallberg B, Palmer RH. Targeting anaplastic lymphoma kinase in neuroblastoma. APMIS. 2019 May;127(5):288-302.

[15] Cheng F, Guo D. MET in glioma: signaling pathways and targeted therapies. J Exp Clin Cancer Res. 2019 Jun 20;38(1):270.

[16] Mulcahy EQX, Colón RR, Abounader R. HGF/MET Signaling in Malignant Brain Tumors. Int J Mol Sci. 2020 Oct 13;21(20):7546.

[17] Nakada M, Kita D, Teng L, Pyko IV, Watanabe T, Hayashi Y, Hamada JI. Receptor Tyrosine Kinases: Principles

and Functions in Glioma Invasion. Adv Exp Med Biol. 2013;986:143-70.

[18] Colavito SA. AXL as a Target in Breast Cancer Therapy. J Oncol. 2020 Feb 14;2020:5291952.

[19] Butti R, Das S, Gunasekaran VP, Yadav AS, Kumar D, Kundu GC. Receptor tyrosine kinases (RTKs) in breast cancer: signaling, therapeutic implications and challenges. Mol Cancer. 2018 Feb 19;17(1):34.

[20] Carter JL, Hege K, Yang J, Kalpage HA, Su Y, Edwards H, Hüttemann M, Taub JW, Ge Y. Targeting multiple signaling pathways: the new approach to acute myeloid leukemia therapy. Signal Transduct Target Ther. 2020 Dec 18;5(1):288.

[21] Tian Z, Niu X, Yao W. Receptor Tyrosine Kinases in Osteosarcoma Treatment: Which Is the Key Target? Front Oncol. 2020 Aug 28;10:1642.

[22] Duan Y, Haybaeck J, Yang Z. Potential of PI3K/AKT/mTOR Pathway in Gastrointestinal Stromal Tumors: Rationale and Progress. Cancers (Basel). 2020 Oct 14;12(10):2972.

[23] Nadhan R, Srinivas P, Pillai MR. RTKs in pathobiology of head and neck cancers. Adv Cancer Res. 2020;147:319-373.

[24] Nelson KN, Peiris MN, Meyer AN, Siari A, Donoghue DJ. Receptor Tyrosine Kinases: Translocation Partners in Hematopoietic Disorders. Trends Mol Med. 2017 Jan;23(1):59-79.

[25] Pacenta HL, Macy ME. Entrectinib and other ALK/TRK inhibitors for the treatment of neuroblastoma. Drug Des Devel Ther. 2018 Oct 23;12:3549-3561.

[26] Al-Salama ZT, Keam SJ. Entrectinib: First Global Approval. Drugs. 2019 Sep;79(13):1477-1483.

[27] Deeks ED. Cabozantinib: A Review in Advanced Hepatocellular Carcinoma. Target Oncol. 2019 Feb;14(1):107-113.

[28] Chabot T, Cheraud Y, Fleury F. Relationships between DNA repair and RTK-mediated signaling pathways. Biochim Biophys Acta Rev Cancer. 2021 Jan;1875(1):188495.

[29] Iida M, Harari PM, Wheeler DL, Toulany M. Targeting AKT/PKB to improve treatment outcomes for solid tumors. Mutat Res. 2020 Jan-Apr; 819-820:111690.

[30] Yamaoka T, Kusumoto S, Ando K, Ohba M, Ohmori T. Receptor Tyrosine Kinase-Targeted Cancer Therapy. Int J Mol Sci. 2018 Nov 6;19(11):3491.

[31] Zhu VW, Klempner SJ, Ou SI. Receptor Tyrosine Kinase Fusions as an Actionable Resistance Mechanism to EGFR TKIs in EGFR-Mutant Non-Small-Cell Lung Cancer. Trends Cancer. 2019 Nov;5(11):677-692.

[32] Wu M, Zhang P. EGFR-mediated autophagy in tumourigenesis and therapeutic resistance. Cancer Lett. 2020 Jan 28;469:207-216.

[33] Altmann DM. Nobel prize-worthy pursuit: cancer immunology and harnessing immunity to tumour neoantigens. Immunology. 2018 Nov;155(3):283-284.

[34] Antony J, Huang RY. AXL-Driven EMT State as a Targetable Conduit in Cancer. Cancer Res. 2017 Jul 15;77(14):3725-3732.

[35] Di Stasi R, De Rosa L, D'Andrea LD. Therapeutic aspects of the Axl/Gas6 molecular system. Drug Discov Today. 2020 Dec;25(12):2130-2148.

[36] Baghy K, Reszegi A, Tátrai P, Kovalszky I. Decorin in the Tumor Microenvironment. Adv Exp Med Biol. 2020;1272:17-38.

[37] Rawla P, Barsouk A, Hadjinicolaou AV, Barsouk A. Immunotherapies and Targeted Therapies in the Treatment of Metastatic Colorectal Cancer. Med Sci (Basel). 2019 Jul 30;7(8):83.

[38] Paranthaman S, Goravinahalli Shivananjegowda M, Mahadev M, Moin A, Hagalavadi Nanjappa S, Nanjaiyah N, Chidambaram SB, Gowda DV. Nanodelivery Systems Targeting Epidermal Growth Factor Receptors for Glioma Management. Pharmaceutics. 2020 Dec 10;12(12):1198.

[39] Merikhian P, Ghadirian R, Farahmand L, Mansouri S, Majidzadeh-A K. MUC1 induces tamoxifen resistance in estrogen receptor-positive breast cancer. Expert Rev Anticancer Ther. 2017 Jul;17(7):607-613.

Chapter 7

The Role of Kinase Inhibitors in Cancer Therapies

Gizem Kursunluoglu, Duygu Erdogan, Elcin Cagatay, Esra Bulut Atalay, Seminay Guler, Yonca Gungor and Hulya Ayar Kayali

Abstract

Protein kinases are enzymes that transfer a phosphate group to the threonine, serine, or tyrosine residues of the target protein, regulating its activity. The activity of these enzymes are very important and strictly regulated in the cell as they promote cell proliferation, survival, and migration. In the case of any dysregulation of these enzymes, they can be associated with cancer initiation and progression. Small-molecule kinase inhibitors approved by the FDA for their improved clinical benefits are currently used in targeted therapy for the treatment of various cancers. So far, there are 62 FDA-approved therapeutic agents targeting different protein kinases, eight of which were approved in 2020. Today, kinase inhibitors are used as FDA approved cancer agents and newly developed ones are evaluated in clinical trials. Those protein kinase inhibitors can be grouped as growth factor receptor inhibitors, Ras/Raf/Mek inhibitors, phosphoinositide 3-kinase (PI3K) and cyclin dependent kinase inhibitors, other targets, and agents such as protein kinase c and 3 phosphoinositide-dependent kinase 1. In this chapter, these kinases, their pathways, and their inhibitors will be discussed in detail.

Keywords: cancer therapy, clinical use, inhibitor, protein kinase, drug

1. Introduction

Protein kinases (PKs) are enzymes that regulate the activity of a protein by adding phosphate group to specific amino acids using ATP as a resource, thereby resulting in a conformational change of that protein. More specifically, they add terminal γ-phosphate group to the serine, threonine or tyrosine residues of the target proteins and this process is called phosphorylation. Phosphorylation of a protein changes its activity, location or downstream function that can result in amplification of the first signal [1]. Furthermore, phosphorylation can also alter biological activities such as transcription and translation. In addition, it can have inhibitory or stimulatory effect on the target. In either case, it has a significant role in regulation of cellular activities.

PK family is one of the largest protein family comprising more than 500 different kinases in the human proteome that is encoded by 2% of the human genome [2]. PKs in regulating protein activity have a massive effect on cell signaling pathways involved in metabolism, immune responses, growth, differentiation, migration, and adaptation.

Because of the potency of PKs, changes in their expression levels or patterns can impact various pathways resulting in disease development including cancers, as well as metabolic and developmental disorders.

PKs are tightly regulated to restrain their potency and any dysregulation could result in a diseased state. Either a kinase itself or the pathway that the kinase is regulated is mutated in many cancers [3–5] and those PKs can be classified as proto-oncogenes. In fact, in 1978, the first identified proto-oncogene encodes a tyrosine kinase called c-Src [6]. Overexpression or dysregulation of oncogenic kinases results in altered signaling pathways and oncogenic transformation. In other words, any perturbation on the regulation of oncogenic kinases can result in anchorage-independent uncontrolled growth and proliferation as well as angiogenesis and metastasis. Exploring the role of kinases in cancer development and progression have highlighted the potential of kinase targeted therapies. In this chapter, we will focus on the kinases' role in oncogenic pathways and the kinase inhibitors targeting these pathways as a therapeutic option.

Protein kinase inhibitors (PKIs) are antineoplastic substances that are used to block the constant or overactivity of dysregulated protein kinases. The first developed PKI called imatinib mesylate (Gleevec, STI571, or CP57148B) targets a fusion protein called "BCR-ABL" which is a constantly active tyrosine kinase that is observed in chronic myeloid leukemia (CML). In addition, imatinib directly inhibits ARG, KIT, and PDGFR tyrosine kinases and used to treat blood neoplasia other than CML and solid tumors that stem from activation of these tyrosine kinases. Consequently, the remarkable success of imatinib had a major impact on researchers to focus on the development of other targeted PKIs that could be potential cancer therapeutics. Following imatinib, other BCL-ABL inhibitors such as nilotinib, dasatinib, bosutinib and ponatinib were developed to overcome imatinib-resistant mutants [7].

The success of imatinib had opened the door to exploration of other oncogenic kinases in other signaling pathways. Those kinase inhibitors can be grouped as growth factor receptor inhibitors, Ras/Raf/Mek inhibitors, phosphoinositide 3-kinase (PI3K) and cyclin dependent kinase inhibitors, other targets and agents such as protein kinase c and 3 phosphoinositide-dependent kinase 1 (PDK1). This chapter will focus on the kinases' role in oncogenic pathways and the kinase inhibitors targeting these pathways as a therapeutic option.

2. Growth factor receptors

Development, growth and homeostasis of multicellular organisms are controlled by growth factors. Growth factors show their activity by binding to their receptors and are required for cell–cell communications for embryonic tissue induction, cell survival, fate determination, apoptosis, cell migration and tissue specialization. These receptors transmit extracellular signals to the intracellular region in two ways: activation of intracellular transporters or direct translocation of the receptor to the nucleus [8].

The feature of cancer is its continuous growth. Growth factors include epidermal growth factor (EGF), vascular endothelial growth factor (VEGF), fibroblast growth factor (FGF), transforming growth factor (TGF), insulin-like growth factor (IGF) and platelet-derived growth factor (PDGF) and they stimulate proliferation, migration and invasion of cancer cell and stromal cell, thereby regulating tumor growth, angiogenesis and metastasis (**Figure 1**) [9]. **Table 1** shows molecules that inhibits growth factor receptors.

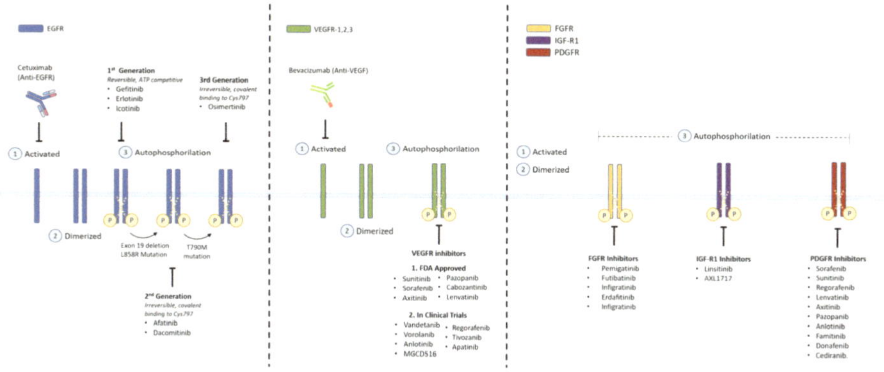

Figure 1.
Kinase inhibitors and their inhibition pathways. Cetuximab binds to EGFR with a higher affinity than EGF and competitively inhibits its binding. Other drugs compete with ATP, inhibits the autophosphorylation process. 1st generation EGFR inhibitors gefitinib, erlotinib and icotinib are not effective against the receptors containing exon 19 deletion and L858R mutations. On the other hand, 3rd generation drug osimertinib is effective against EGFR containing exon 19 deletion, L858R and T790M mutations. Bevacizumab binds to VEGFR ligand VEGF, inhibiting its binding with VEGFR. Other inhibitors of VEGFR, FGFR, IGF-R1 and PDGFR target autophosphorylation mechanism, thereby prohibiting the downstream activation of other proteins.

2.1 Epidermal growth factor receptor

One of the most studied drugs in human cancer is the EGF family of receptor tyrosine kinases (RTKs), also called ErbB or HER receptors [8]. Family of EGF receptor (EGFR) comprises four receptor proteins: ErbB-1/EGFR-1 to −4 (also called HER 1–4). These proteins are expressed on cell surface and have alike structure: an intracellular domain with kinase activity, a transmembrane domain and an extracellular domain with ligand binding site [10]. The binding of EGFR ligand initiates homo- and heterodimers between receptors, activating cascades of mitogenic and anti-apoptotic signal [11].

The dimerization is required to activate the intracellular tyrosine kinase domain and C-terminal tail phosphorylation. Its autophosphorylation then promotes either directly or by adaptor proteins, the signal transduction pathways including Ras/MAPK, PI(3)kinase/Akt, PLCg1/PKC, and STAT pathways [8] in modulating differentiation, cellular proliferation, and survival [11].

EGFR has been extensively studied for cancer therapeutics due to mutations, deletions, and overexpression in tumors [11]. EGFR is generally investigated in non-small cell lung cancer (NSCLC): its amplification is ~80% and its mutation is 20% [12, 13]. When compared to chemotherapy used in NSCLC patients, EGFR TKIs have more than twice the progression-free survival (PFS) with actionable mutations of EGFR. Moreover, they have better objective response rates (ORRs), response time, life quality, and reduction in treatment- associated toxicity [14]. First generation EGFR-tyrosine kinase inhibitors (TKIs) bind reversibly to EGFR and block ATP-TK domain binding and this blockage causes cell death by inhibiting cell proliferation [15]. Some examples of these EGFR-TKIs are gefitinib, erlotinib, and icotinib [14]. When looked at the second-generation EGFR-TKIs these irreversibly bind to EGFR. Afatinib and dacomitinib can be given examples as second generation [14]. Although dacomitinib has improved median PFS, hazard ratio, and median overall survival [16, 17] compared to first-line treatment, the usage of afatinib and dacomitinib in clinical practice may be limited due to having increased toxicities [18].

EGFR T790M mutation causes almost 50% resistance to EGFR-TKIs of first and second generations [19]. As an EGFR TKI of third-generation, osimertinib inhibits

Target	Inhibitors			
EGFR	**Gefitinib** 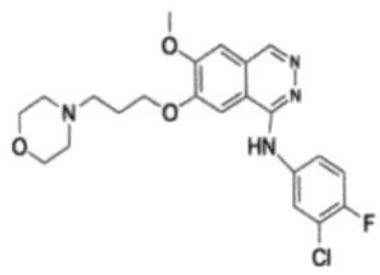	**Erlotinib** 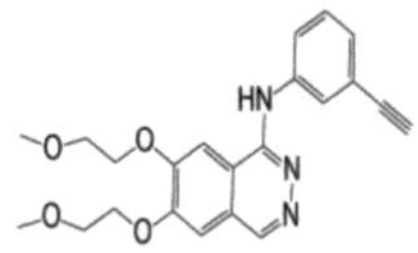	**Icotinib** 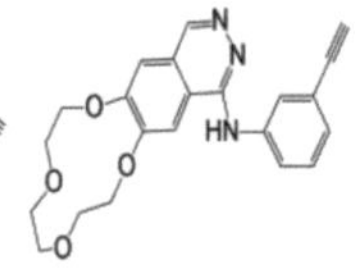	
	Dacomitinib 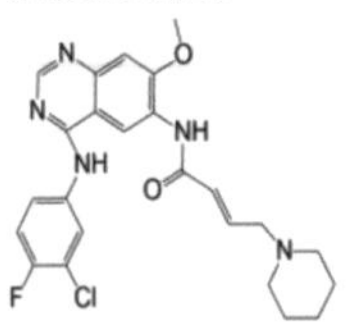	**Osimertinib** 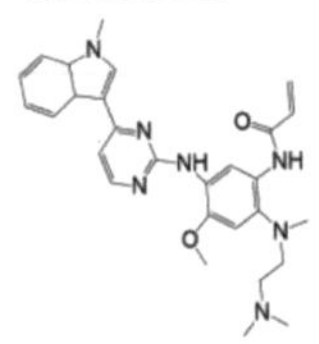	**Almonertinib** 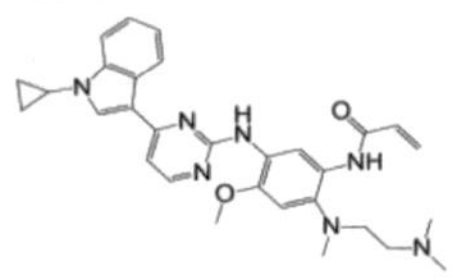	
	Furmonertinib 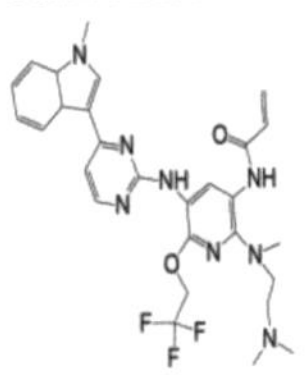	**Rezivertinib (BPI-7711)** 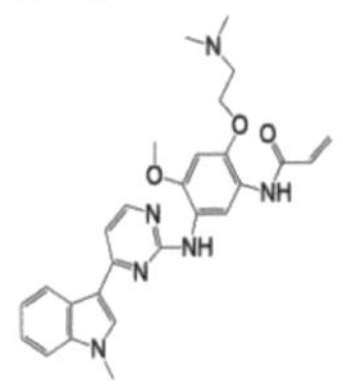	**Lazertinib** 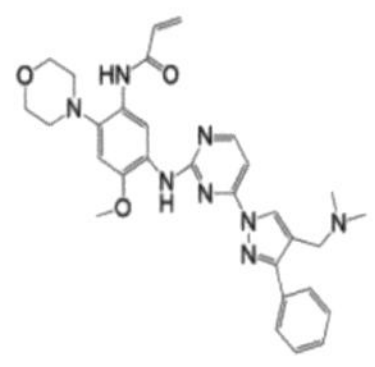	**Nazartinib** 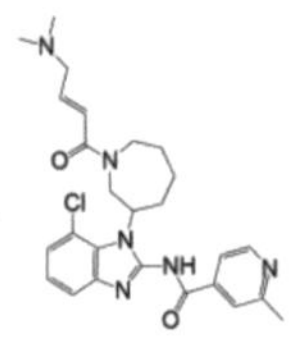
VEGFR and PDGFR	**Sunitinib** 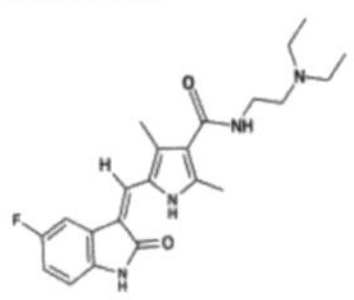	**Sorafenib** 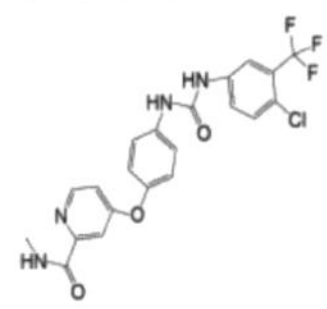	**Axitinib** 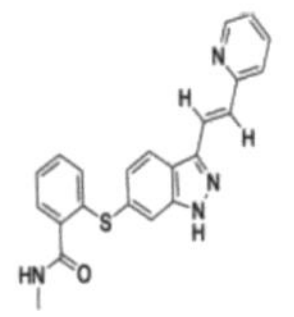	**Pazopanib** 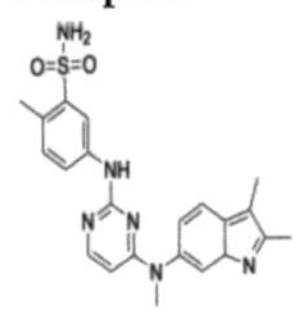
	Lenvatinib 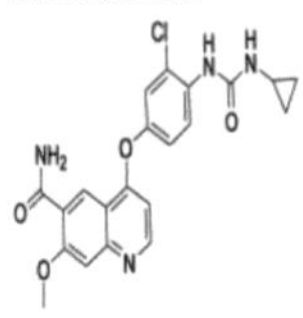	**Anlotinib** 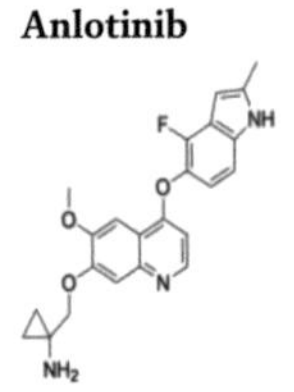	**Regorafenib** 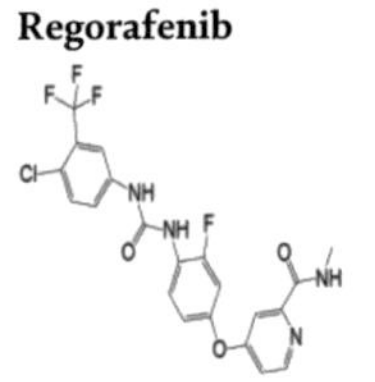	**Donafenib** 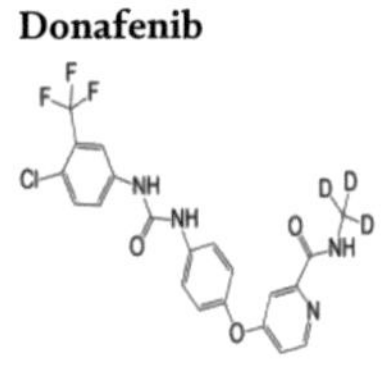
VEGFR	**Cabozantinib** 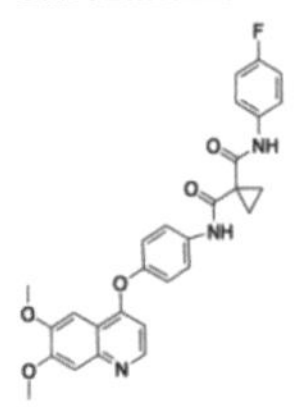	**Vandetanib** 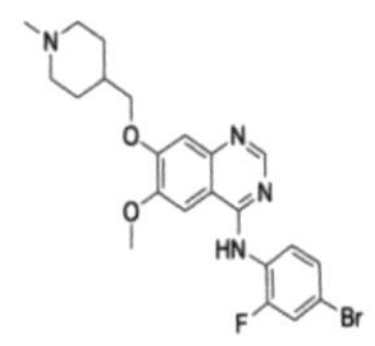	**Vorolanib** 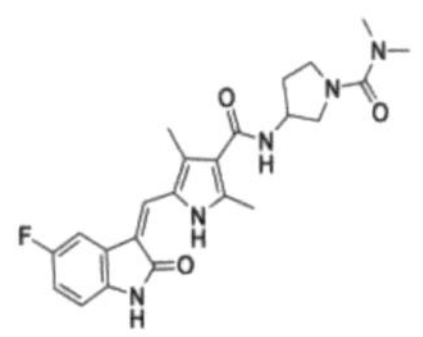	
	Apatinib 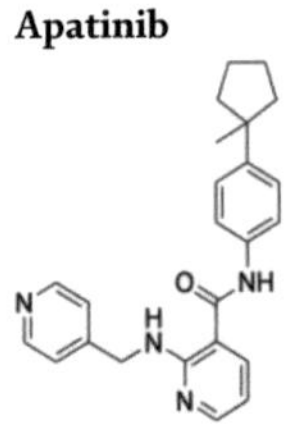	**Sitravatinib (MGCD516)** 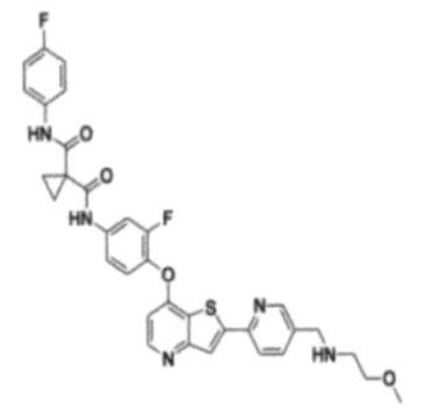	**Tivozanib** 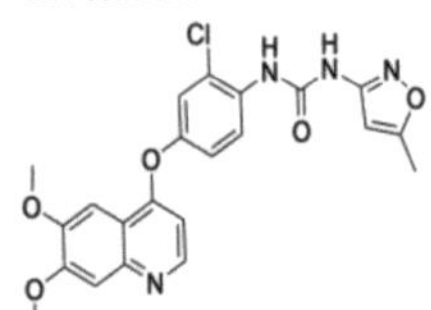	

Target	Inhibitors		
FGFR	**Futibatinib** 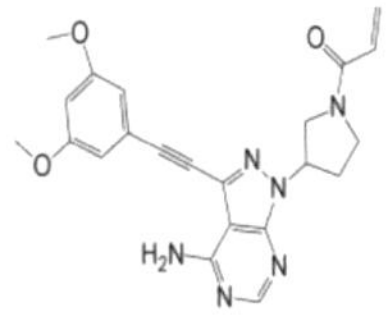	**Infigratinib** 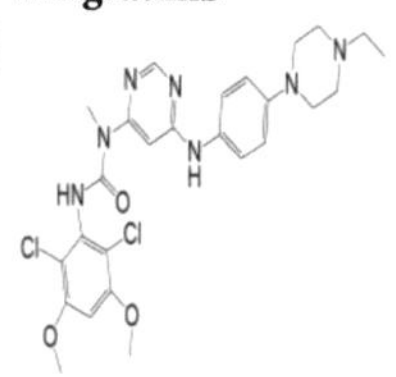	**Erdafitinib** 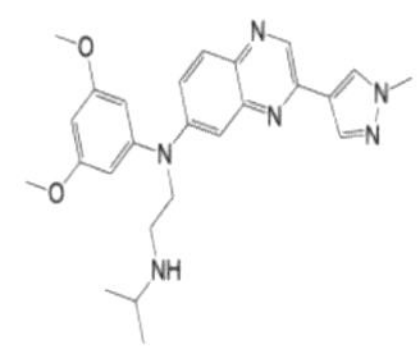
TGF-βR	**Galunisertib** 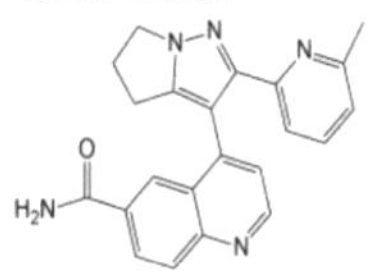		**LY2109761** 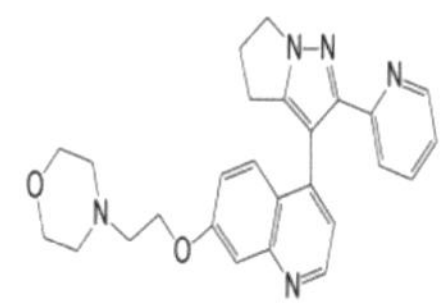
IGFR	**Linsitinib** 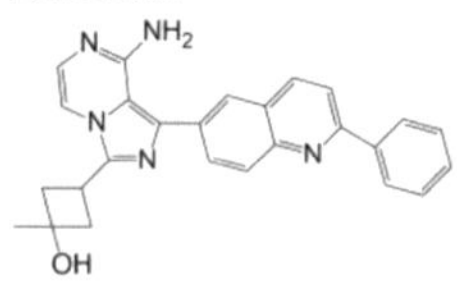		**Picropodophyllin** (AXL1717) 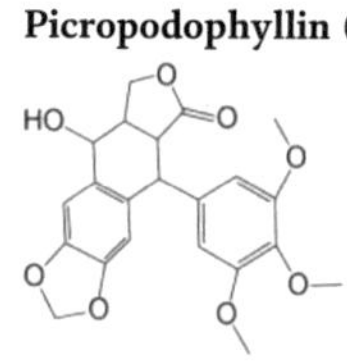
PDGFR	**Famitinib** 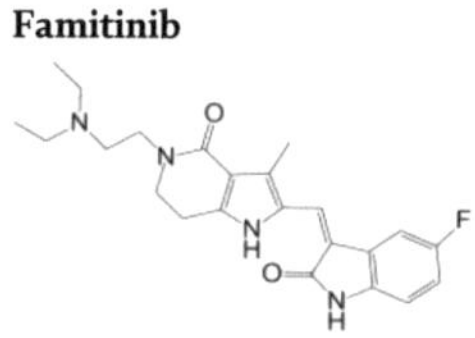		**Cediranib** 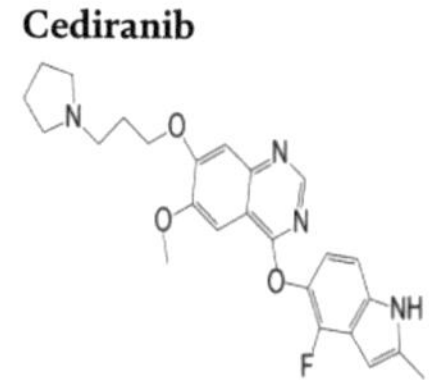

Table 1.
Structures of growth factor receptors inhibitors.

both EGFR T790M mutations and EGFR-sensitizing [20] and it is promising for central nervous system (CNS) metastatic patients which is due to EGFR mutation in NSCLC patients [20] or after treatment with EGFR-TKIs of first- or second-generation [21]. Other EGFR TKIs as a third-generation for advanced NSCLC with mutation in EGFR T790M are almonertinib [22], furmonertinib (AST2818) [23], BPI-7711 [24], lazertinib (YH25448) [25], and nazartinib (EGF816) [26], and they have exhibited acceptable safeties and promising efficacies. Almonertinib was also approved by China National Medical Products Administration (NMPA).

Monoclonal antibodies (mAbs), cetuximab and panitumumab, have been used against EGFR and are approved for metastatic colorectal cancer (CRC) treatment. Only small patient subgroups to cetuximab and panitumumab indicate clinical benefit. The best response to cetuximab and panitumumab is seen in patients with the combination of wild type KRAS, BRAF, and PIK3CA and PTEN protein express [27]. Trastuzumab is another mAb used in EGFR/HER2 pathway for the treatment of HER2-positive breast cancers [28].

2.2 Vascular endothelial growth factor receptor

Vascular endothelial growth factors (VEGF) are a family of polypeptides contain highly conserved receptor binding domain in disulfide-node [29]. There are two types of VEGF; VEGF-A and VEGF-B, which bind their receptors named RTK. VEGF members display plural interactions with RTKs are the critical factors for blood vessel formation which cause cord formation and tubulogenesis, differentiation of endothelial cells, proliferation, migration. In mammals, the vascular endothelial growth factor receptor (VEGFR), transmembrane tyrosine kinase receptors, comprises three members VEGFR-1 (Flt-1), VEGFR-2 (KDR/Flk-1) and VEGFR-3 (Flt-4), and control the generation of blood and lymphatic vessels [30].

VEGFRs have seven immunoglobulin (Ig)-like domains on the extracellular site and two split tyrosine kinase domains in the intracellular site [10]. In adults, while the vascular endothelial cells are posess largely VEGFR-1 and VEGFR-2 in their structure, the lymphatic endothelial cells have VEGFR-3 [31]. The literature shows that VEGF pathway is critical for renal cell carcinoma (RCC) initiation and progression, and VEGFRs targeted TKIs have been used for most favorable RCC treatment strategy.

In recent years, VEGFR-associated multi-targeted TKIs have been revealed as anti-tumor agents for cancer treatment [18]. VEGFR-targeted therapeutic agents have become the main element used for RCC patients treatment [31]. The FDA has approved 6 small molecules, named as sunitinib, sorafenib, axitinib, pazopanib, cabozantinib and lenvatinib, that inhibit VEGFR1/2/3 for use in RCC treatment. Additionally, for clinical trials, seven VEGFR inhibitors; vandetanib, vorolanib, anlotinib, MGCD516, regorafenib, tivozanib, and apatinib are under review [31].

Not only VEGFRs targeted and block by these drugs, also some other receptors generally overexpressed in RCC, platelet-derived growth factor (PDGF) receptors a and b (PDGFR-a/b), stem cell factor receptor (c-KIT), FMS-like tyrosine kinase-3 (FLT3), tyrosine protein kinase MET, rearranged during transfection (RET), tyrosine kinase that contains immunoglobulin-like loops and epidermal growth factor-similar domains-2 (Tie2), fibroblast growth factor receptor (FGFR), the GAS6 receptor (AXL), serine/threonine protein kinase Raf-1, colony stimulating factor1 receptor (CSF1R), and discoidin domain receptor (DDR) targeted by these small drugs. In addition, growth, proliferation and angiogenesis of tumor cells are significantly inhibited by the effects of VEGFR1/2/3 inhibitors. The humanized IgG1 monoclonal antibody approved in 2009, Bevacizumab can bind VEGF and for use in first-line therapy for RCC in combination with IFN-α [32].

Besides, in hepatocellular carcinoma (HCC), the efficiency of VEGFR-associated multi-targeted TKIs was demonstrated. Especially Sorafenib can target VEGFR, PDGFR, FGFR, and other signaling targets and prefered as first line therapy in inoperable cases [33, 34]. In phase II/III studies of Donafenib, VEGFR-associated multitargeted TKI, is shown a higher overall survival rate than sorafenib in advanced HCC cases [35]. Moreover, regorafenib [36], apatinib [37] and cabozantinib [38] are used for second-line treatment of HCC. More recently, it is shown that Pembrolizumab is anti programmed cell death protein-1 (PD-1) antibody and lenvatinib combination therapies demonstrated promising anti-tumor effect on untreated/inoperable HCC patients and this combination named as breakthrough therapy by FDA [39].

For lung cancer therapy (on NSCLC [40] and SCLC [41]), Anlotinib showed promising results and was approved for further-line therapy by(National Medical Products Administration of China (NMPA) [18]. Furthermore, similar results identified in thyroid carcinoma and soft tissue sarcoma (STS) patients [42].

2.3 Fibroblast growth factor receptor

Fibroblast growth factor receptors (FGFRs), which are members of receptor tyrosine kinase can be thought as single pass membrane proteins due to the cellular membrane covering in a single region [43]. There are four transmembrane proteins (FGFR1–4) for the FGFR family and different isoforms of them with changed ligand specificity [10]. Upon binding of the different FGF ligands to different FGF receptors, auto-phosphorylation and kinase activation are initiated by FGFR dimerization. This binding causes cell death inhibition and uncontrolled growth, respectively due to downstream anti-apoptotic PI3K/AKT signals and mitogenic growth signals (MAPK) so the interaction FGF-FGFR plays a critical role in tumorigenesis. Moreover, the downstream of PLC/PKC pathway joins the MAPK pathway to promote cell growth [10].

The use of FGFR pathway downstream molecules as targets in anti-cancer drugs has attracted attention, and these drugs are small compounds and antibodies against cancer driver mutations in FGFRs and related signaling molecules [43]. Most FGFR-TKIs belong to multiple target TKIs [18].

FGFR2 changes are associated with the cholangiocarcinoma (CCA). Pemigatinib, a FGFR1–3 TKI, has been accepted for the treatment of locally advanced or metastatic CCA [44]. Some other FGFR-TKIs (such as futibatinib, infigratinib) also have the potential to be used for CCA based on their results [45].

In addition to CCA, FGFR2 changes also play a role in urothelial carcinoma (UC). Fusions and mutations in FGFR2/3 are seen in 20% of patients with UC [46]. Treatment with erdafitinib, a FGFR1–4 TKI, has been accepted for the adult patients with previously treated metastatic or locally advanced FGFR2/3-mutated UC. Response was more promising as second-line therapy for advanced UC compared to antibody-drug conjugates such as enfortumab vedotin or sacituzumab govitecan [47] and pembrolizumab [48]. In addition, other inhibitors of pan-FGFR are investigated and for example infigratinib (BGJ 398) is examined in the treatment of UC holding a FGFR3 mutation [47].

2.4 Transforming growth factor-β receptor

Transforming growth factor-beta (TGF-β) is a cytokine which has different functions and modulates cell growth and differentiation, extracellular matrix production, apoptosis, angiogenesis, cell motility, and cellular immune responses. Interestingly, TGF- β shows different effects on tumorigenesis. Although it acts as a tumor suppressor in the early stages, it advances tumor growth by producing a more suitable environment for tumor invasion and metastasis in later stages [49].

There are three membrane receptors for the TGF-β receptor (TGF-βR) family: TβRI, TβRII and TβRIII. Their expression in various cell types control different cellular functions by altering signals upon ligand binding of TGF-β [10]. When high binding affinity is established between activated TGF-β and TβRII signaling is started. The binding needs altering the conformation of TβRII by engagement of TβRIII [49]. Receptors transphosphorylation is triggered after binding is created between TGF-β ligand and transmembrane receptor serine/threonine kinase (type I and II) complex. After that, SMAD proteins in C-terminal serine are phosphorylated by activated receptors. SMAD complexes which are activated control target genes transcription by migrating to the nucleus [50], thereby controlling cell proliferation, migration, survival, and differentiation [10].

TGF-β can signal via intracellular Smad proteins and some Smad independent pathways involving ERK, MAP kinase, PI3K, JNK, p38, and AKT [49]. The Smad pathway is very important in the antiproliferative properties of TGF-β and modifications in the Smad system by missense mutations [51, 52]. Moreover, blocking of the phosphorylation process or Smad 2/3 complex formation has been demonstrated to be effective in tumor development [53]. The TGF-β overexpression has been determined in many tumors containing cancers of the breast, colon, liver, stomach, lung, esophagus, kidney, prostate, pancreas, brain, and malignant melanoma, as well as certain hematological malignancies [54–61]. Some small-molecule TKIs of TβR II and TβR III can block the signaling pathway of TGF-β-mediated receptor.

Galunisertib (LY2157299) monohydrate has shown powerful as a TβR I inhibitor by reducing Smad2 phosphorylation in pancreatic, colorectal cancer, lung cancer [62] and ovarian cancer [63]. LY2157299 is another promising inhibitor of Smad2 phosphorylation for hepatocellular carcinoma models [64]. It moved to Phase II and was approved by the FDA for liver cancer as an orphan drug in 2013. LY2109761 for metastatic NSCLC [65], colorectal cancer [66] could also investigated as a kinase inhibitor. In addition, Ki26894 blocks Smad2 phosphorylation by binding to the TβR I-ATP domain and its activity was demonstrated in breast cancer [67] and gastric cancer [68].

2.5 Insuline-like growth factor receptor

The insulin-like growth factor receptor (IGFR) family includes two cell membrane receptors, named as IGF-IR and IGF-IIR. IGF-IR (that also forms a heterodimer with the insulin receptor [IR]) has higher affinity to insulin-like growth factor 1 (IGF-I) but IGF-II comparatively has lower affinity. Although IGF-IR, receptor tyrosine kinase, has the triggering effects on IGF-I and IGF-II and thus on cell proliferation, migration and invasion, IGF-IIR lacks kinase activity [9].

Pathways activated by the presence of IGF and progressive pathological and physiological processes take place through proper receptors, named as IGFR. The mature IGF-IR have homodimer structure, containing α2 and β2 chains bounded with disulfide bonds. The intracellular domain is autophosphorylated by the binding of ligands and the downstream processes continue with the activation of a number of proteins. In several carcinomas, proliferation, transformation and metastasis are induced by overexpression of IGFIR genes. IGF-IIR, called mannose-6 phosphate receptor, M6P, is formed as a single polypeptide chain and performs as a "scavenger receptor" that suppresses tumor growth, modulates invasiveness, and blocks angiogenesis. Mutated IGFIIR locus could be found in lung cells and early phase hepatocellular carcinoma [10].

Especially, cancer associated macrophages, tumor cells and liver cells secrete IGF. The increased risk of breast and prostate cancer is correlated with high levels of IGF in the circulating system [69, 70]. For smokers,there is a moderate correlation between IGF level and lung cancer risk [71]. IGF-I is not related to colorectal cancer but takes increased risk for colorectal cancer [72]. Multiple signaling pathways of PI3K/Akt, JAK/STAT, MAPK, Src and focal adhesion kinase (FAK) lead to the proliferation, survival, and migration of cancer cells by binding IGF to its appropriate receptor, are activated.

In many human tumors, especially mesenchymal, epithelial and hematopoietic cancers, the growth of cancer cells, metastasis and the formation of drug resistance can be associated with the activation of IGF signaling pathways [73–75].

The IGF-IR has been evaluated as a target protein in cancer treatment. There are some small-molecule inhibitors and anti-IGF-IR mAbs used in pre-clinical models and clinical trials. A dual IGF-IR/Insulin receptor inhibitor, linsitinib (OSI-906), is investigated in phase II in recurrent small cell lung cancer patients. However, clinical activity failed to show improvement in small cell lung cancer, metastatic or advanced adrenocortical carcinoma, metastatic colorectal cancer, advanced NSLC, gastrointestinal stromal tumors and metastatic prostate cancer. AXL1717 is studied in early phase with relapsed malignant astrocytomas and can show long-term stable disease and patients' survival [9].

2.6 Platelet derived growth factor receptor

Platelets produce platelet-derived growth factor (PDGF) and are secreted from both epithelial and mesenchymal cells [76]. The PDGF family has five isoforms (PDGF AA, BB, AB, CC, and DD) that bind to two RTKs, PDGFRα and PDGFRβ. After activation of PDGFRα and β, they promote cell proliferation, migration and survival through initiating signaling pathway with the inclusion of the extracellular signal-regulated kinase 1/2 (ERK) and phosphatidylinositol 3-kinase (PI3K)/AKT [77].

Overexpressed platelet-derived growth factor receptor (PDGFR) is associated with the formation of various human tumors like glioma, neurofibroma, ovarian cancer, prostate cancer, and non-small cell lung carcinoma. In addition, PDGF accelerates angiogenesis by increasing VEGF expression and development of cancer-related fibroblasts that directly or indirectly affect tumor formation. Moreover, PDGF plays a role in gene amplification [76].

To enhance anti-angiogenesis effect and suppress tumor growth PDGFR is targeted by most VEGFR-related multiple kinase inhibitors such as sorafenib, sunitinib, regorafenib, lenvatinib, axitinib, pazopanib, anlotinib, famitinib, donafenib and cediranib. These inhibitors can be critical to treat various cancer types [18].

3. Ras/Raf/MEK pathway inhibitors

Ras/Raf/MEK pathway inhibitors are important as kinase inhibitors in various cancer treatment. Firstly, the Ras protein known as Ras GTP-binding protein is the member of small G protein family, which has an important role in transmitting growth factor and relay signals from activated growth factor receptors (GFR) (**Figure 2**).

Ras proteins are regulated by a GDP-GTP cycle, different form is carried out when bound to GDP or GTP, inactive form is Ras-GDP and active form is Ras-GTP [78]. Therefore this cycle has been stimulated via receptor activation then Ras proteins bind to GTP (active form), cellular proliferation and other effects are

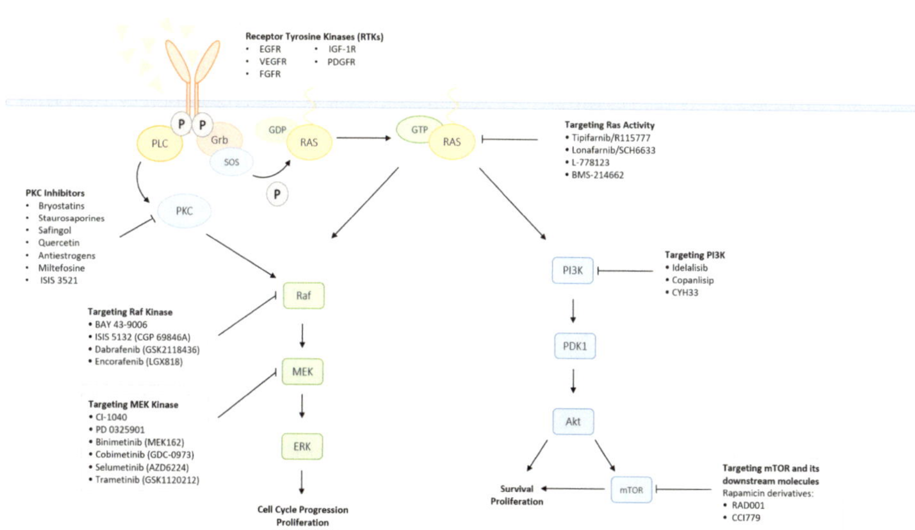

Figure 2.
Downstream molecular pathways that are activated upon stimulation of receptor tyrosine kinases (RTKs). The main pathways include protein kinase C (PKC), Ras–Raf–Mek and PI3K pathways.

promoted [79]. Ras protein associate with cell transformation such as cell growth, differentiation, apoptosis, cell migration, this Ras regulation is carried out by modulating some signaling molecules by translocating them to the plasma membrane for activation. Since Ras proteins play critical role as a branch point in signal transduction and orchestrate the activity of multiple signaling pathways such as Raf/MEK/ERK [78].

Numerous of the signal transduction pathways are occurred through protein kinases regulating of cellular metabolism [80]. One of the most important key protein kinases are Ras, Raf and MEK for targeting of the anticancer drug and also, Ras mutations are quite common as they are identified in about 30% of cancers [81–83]. Ras protein activations are depended on the cancer type, for instance N-Ras in lymphoid and myeloid cancers, K-Ras in colon and pancreatic cancers, H-Ras in bladder and kidney cancers [84]. One of the main reasons for this situation is thought to be the disorder in protein kinase activity. Thus, the protein kinase enzyme family is seen as one of the most important drug targets of the 21st century in many diseases, especially cancer, and there are 62 FDA-approved therapeutic agents targeting different protein kinases, eight of which were approved in 2020 [85]. Thus, today, kinase inhibitors are both used as FDA approved cancer agents and evaluated in clinical trials. Protein kinase inhibitors related to the Ras / Raf / MEK pathway, which is the subject of this part, are structurally classified as small molecules and antisense oligonucleotides and structure of Ras/Raf/MEK kinase inhibitors is shown in **Table 2**.

3.1 Ras kinase inhibitors

Ras protein, which has the ability to induce different growth and proliferation pathways of the cell, is located in the cell membrane. And most importantly, overactivation of mutated Ras can induce to make progress in cancer. Farnesyl Transferase enzyme catalyzes the first step of the reaction in the posttranslational modification of both the normal and mutated Ras gene, thus it is easier to settle on the cell membrane. FTase, one of the tansferase enzymes, targets Ras proteins, adding a farnesyl group to it. After the essential transfer step, the activity of the Ras protein has been inhibited by Ftase [86, 87]. Therefore, FTase enzyme and the downstream pathways of the Ras protein are considered to be one of the most important groups of targets that can be medicated in cancer therapy [88]. The potential anti-cancer agent effect of Farnesyl Transferase inhibitors acting as kinase inhibitors which is affecting Ras and Ras downstream will be reviewed in this part. Various FTase inhibitors such as tipifarnib/R115777, lonafarnib/SCH66336, L-778123 and BMS-214662 have been used primarily in clinical trials and phase studies [89].

The antitumor activity of tipifarnib, a potent and selective farnesyltransferase inhibitor, also known as R115777, has been evaluated the antiproliferative effect of tipifarnib, 53 human tumor cell lines have been studied and 75% were obtained to be sensitive to R115777 [90, 91]. The strong potency effect of Tipifarnib was detected in SU86.86 human pancreatic cells, CAPAN-2 human pancreatic cells and NCI-H441 human lung cells and these cells espacially include the KRAS 12 mutation cells [90, 91]. Tipifarnib has been studied as a phase 2 study on 249 adult patients with refractory urothelial carcinoma (UC) and HRAS mutation. This study shows that tipifarnib is effective in previously treated metastatic UC patients by inhibiting the processing of newly synthesized proteins [92]. In refractory advanced colorectal cancer as a Phase III study, it had an acceptable toxicity profile and was well tolerated but did not improve overall survival according to the best supportive [93], and R115777 was not effective in metastatic colorectal cancer patients in another Phase II study [94]. Another phase two studies of R115777 emphazied that

Target	Inhibitors		
Ras Kinase	**Tipifarnib (R115777)** 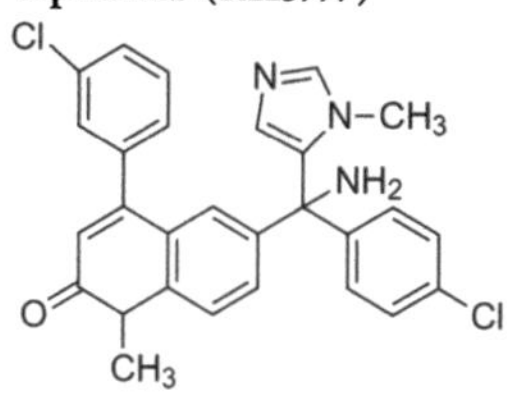		**Lonafarnib (SCH66336)** 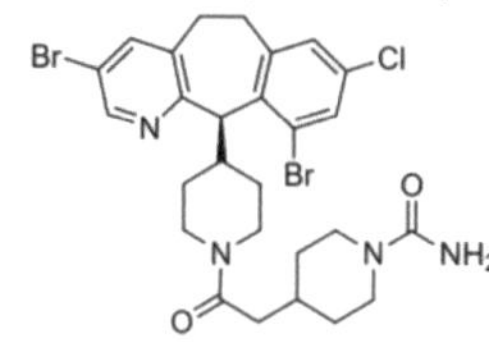
	L-778123 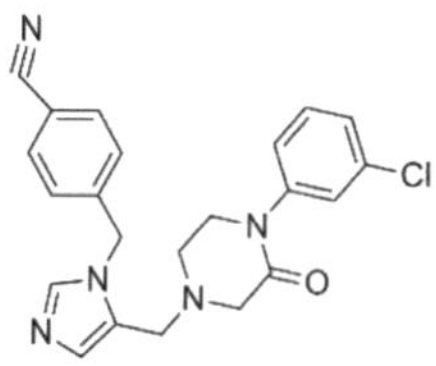		**BMS-214662** 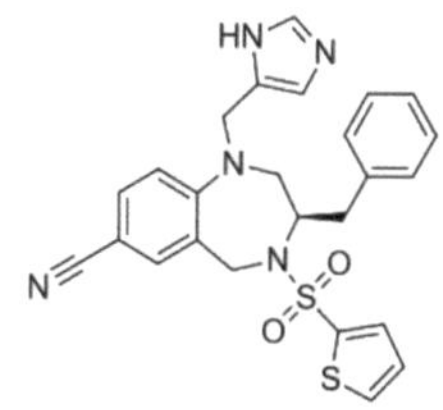
Raf Kinase	**Encorafenib (LGX818)** 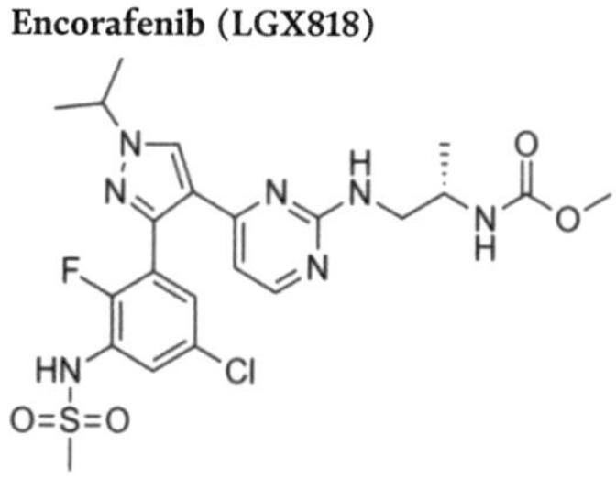		**Dabrafenib (GSK2118436)** 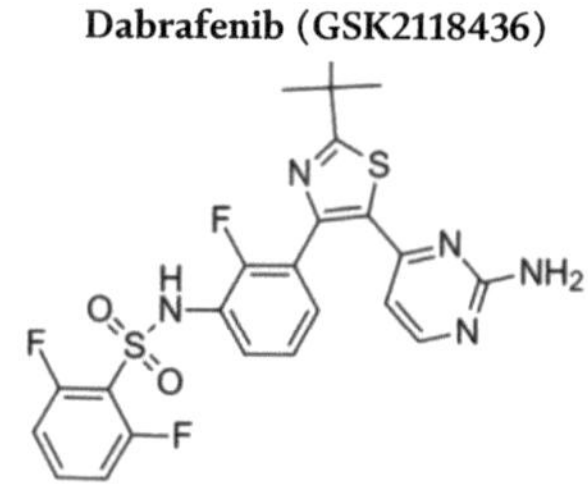
		BAY 43-9006 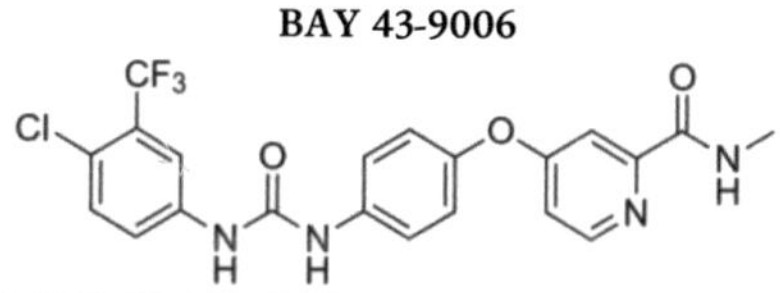	
MEK Kinase	**CI-1040** 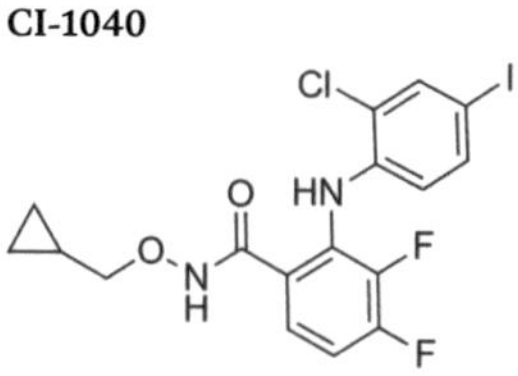	**Binimetinib (MEK162)** 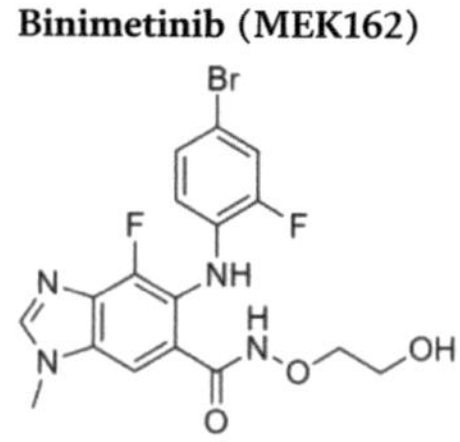	**PD 0325901** 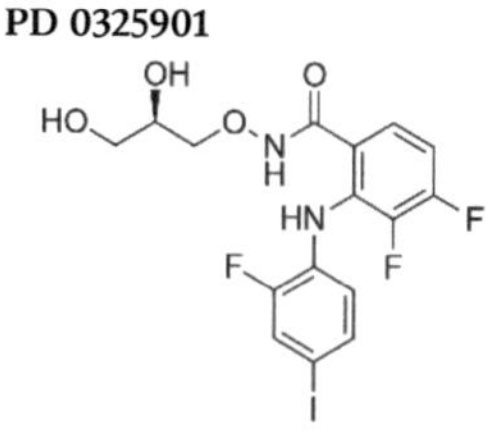
	Cobimetinib (GDC-0973) 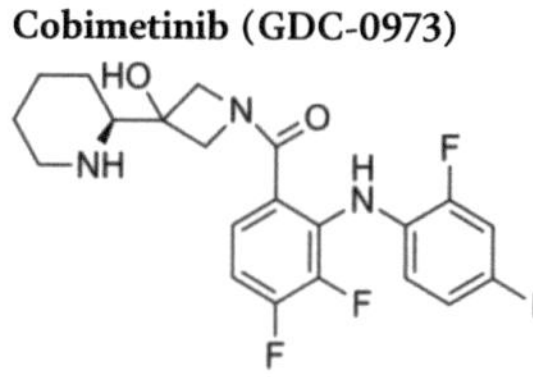	**Selumetinib (AZD6224)** 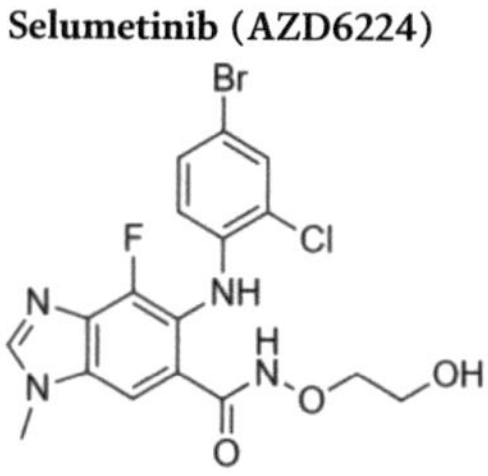	**Trametinib (GSK1120212)** 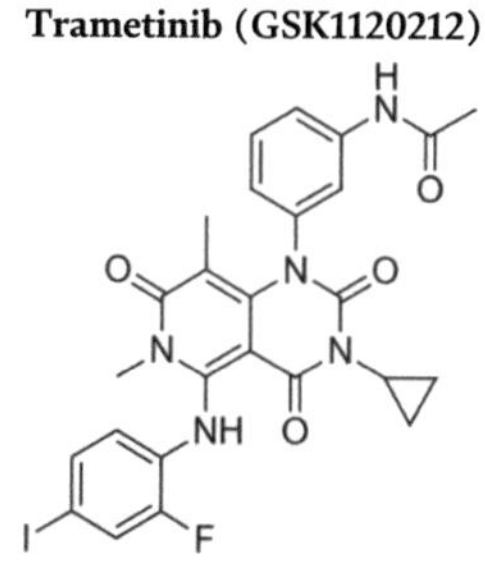

Table 2.
Structures of Ras–Raf–MEK kinase inhibitors.

antitumor properties were not observed in metastatic c pancreatic cancer and did not improve overall survival in advanced non-small cell lung cancer [95, 96]. Farnesyl transferase inhibitor R115777, one of the protein kinase inhibitors, which are thought to be effective in the Ras pathway, has being continuing to be evaluated different combination therapies studies as well as single therapy [97].

Lonafarnib (SCH66336) as a clinical candidate FTase inhibitor, showed antitumor activity in vivo lung, colon, pancreas, bladder and prostate human tumor xenograft models [98]. Various antiproliferative effects of the SCH66336 agent were observed in eight human astrocytoma cell lines with different concentrations of IC50 values (0.6 mM - 32.3 mM) [99]. Growth inhibitory effects of the drug SCH66336 were observed in human tumor xenografts with various tumor models (colon, lung, pancreatic, prostatic carcinoma and a H-ras transgenic mouse model) [100]. In the other phase 2 studies, Lonafarnib, which was used as a combined treatment with paclitaxel, had clinical benefit and low toxicity in patients with non-small cell lung carcinoma, while the targeted response of Lonafarnib was not observed in 5-fluorouracil and irinotecan-resistant metastatic colorectal cancer and gastrointestinal toxicity was observed in single therapy [97] .

L-778123, a peptidomimetic farnesyl protein transferase (FPTase) inhibitor, was administered to patients with solid malignancies developed in phase 1 studies and their toxicity levels were investigated. While unacceptable toxicity was observed at the doses of L-778123 given as 1120 mg / m2 / day, the dose of 560 mg/m2/day was well tolerated. Also, no objective tumor response was observed following drug administration in this phase 1 study [101]. When the toxicity of L-778123 and radiotherapy combination was evaluated in phase 1 studies, it was found to be at an acceptable level in pancreatic cancer patients [102]. Although there are no important studies on cancer treatment in phase 1, this drug has been stopped in its clinical development due to its severe and unexpected toxicity [103].

3.2 Raf kinase inhibitors

Receptor tyrosine kinase effector Raf derives its name from "Rapidly Accelerated Fibrosarcoma" [104]. There are 3 different isoforms of Raf family related to serine/threonine protein kinases, namely Raf-1, A-Raf and B-Raf [105]. Critical steps are needed for Raf activation to occur, these are Raf-1 phosphorylation, binding of Raf protein to Ras-GTP, oligomerization of Raf protein, interaction of Raf protein with membrane lipids, and conformational changes in Ras-induced Raf protein [106]. Phosphorylation of Raf kinases plays an important role in cell cycle regulation, proliferation and differentiation, cell survival, apoptosis, and many cellular processes [107]. Furthermore, Raf kinase isoforms become overactive in a variety of solid tumors such as renal cell carcinoma (RCC), hepatocellular carcinoma (HCC), non-small cell lung cancer (NSCLC), and papillary thyroid carcinoma. BAY 43–9006 is a potent Raf kinase inhibitor with significant activity in four different types of human tumors, including colon, pancreatic, lung and ovarian tumors. The in vivo study of BAY 43–9006 shows that after 14 days of injection, tumor growth is strongly suppressed in athymic mice modeled with human tumors [107]. It suggests that BAY 43–9006 may have clinical potential as a cancer therapeutic agent with a new mechanism of action with its antitumor activity [107]. One of the other important raf kinase inhibitors is ISIS 5132 (CGP 69846A), for which phase I and II studies have also been performed. This Raf kinase inhibitor provides inhibition of c-Raf mRNA expression and inhibits the proliferation of lung, colon, cervical, prostate and ovarian carcinoma cell lines [105]. According to the phase1 and phase 2 studies performed with ISIS 5132, no significant response occurred in small cell or non-small cell lung carcinoma, hormone-resistant prostate cancer, and Colorectal cancer [105]. There are two FDA approved molecules among Raf Kinase Inhibitors, one of which is Dabrafenib (GSK2118436), which is effective in $BRAF^{V600E/K}$ melanomas, $BRAF^{V600E}$ NSCLC, $BRAF^{V600E}$ anaplastic thyroid cancers, and Encorafenib (LGX818), which is suitable for combination therapy with binimetinib for BRAF$^{V600E/K}$ melanomas [85].

3.3 MEK kinase inhibitors

One of the most important involved in cancer biology downstream targets of Ras is mitogen activated extracellular signal regulated kinase (MEK) [108]. Various MEK inhibitors, one of the first selective inhibitors of mitogen-activated protein kinase (MAPK) pathway activation, were investigated in phase 1 and 2 studies [109]. CI-1040, the first MEK inhibitor participating in the clinical study, was tested on 66 patients, while a partial response was observed in one patient with pancreatic cancer, stable disease was observed in 19 patients with various solid tumors such as non-small cell lung, breast and colon cancer [110]. PD 0325901, a second generation MEK inhibitor, was studied in 27 patients, while a partial response was observed in two patients with melanoma, and stable disease was observed in eight patients with various solid tumors [111]. There are 4 different FDA approved small molecule protein kinase inhibitors, for which "MEK1/2" is the primary target. These FDA approved MEK protein kinase inhibitors, Binimetinib (MEK162), Cobimetinib (GDC-0973), Selumetinib (AZD6224), Trametinib (GSK1120212), are respectively effective in these diseases; Combination therapy with encorafenib for BRAF$^{V600E/K}$ melanomas, melanomas in combination with vemurafenib, Neurofibromatosis type I, BRAFV$^{600E/K}$ melanomas, BRAF^{V600E} NSCLC [85].

4. Phosphoinositide 3-kinase (PI3K) pathway inhibitors

The activation of PI3K, a superfamily of lipid kinases, leads to the production of lipid seconder molecule phosphatidylinositol-3,4,5-trisphosphate (PIP3) which recruits phosphatidylinositide-dependent protein kinase (PDK1) and Akt protein kinases to the plasma membrane. Akt that activated and phosphorylated from PDK1 and mTOR, phosphorylates several target proteins either at the plasma membrane or in the cytosol and nucleus (**Figure 2**). Cell proliferation controlled by the PI3K pathway is partially dependent on a large kinase protein called mammalian target of rapamycin (mTOR). mTOR complex 1 plays a role in cell growth and survival by stimulating nutrient uptake and metabolism. Akt activates mTOR independently of phosphorylation at complex 1 [112].

PI3K has three different classes (I, II and III) and four different isoforms (α, β, γ, δ). While it has central physiological roles in cancer, diabetes, and aging, the isoform within each class has distinct roles.Several small molecules have been produced with good pharmacological properties that have been tested in various cancers to selectively inhibit PI3K, AKT or, mTOR [113].

Idelalisib and Copanlisip are FDA-approved drugs. Idelalisib has been selectively developed for the delta isoform of PI3K p110 inhibitor. This purine-quinazoline derivative has been used for the treatment of patients with CLL, relapsed follicular B-cell non-Hodgkin lymphoma (NHL), and relapsed small lymphocytic leukemia (SLL) [114]. The combination study with rituximab resulted in a significant increase in the response rate and overall survival on CLL patients [115]. Copanlisip is the inhibitor of the pan-class I PI3K, which shows preferential activity against p110α and p110δ as compared with p110β and p110γ. It has been used for the treatment of various subtypes of indolent and aggressive malignant lymphoma such as NHL, relapsed follicular lymphoma (FL), and CLL in phase II study. This small molecule, administered intravenously, becomes advantageous compared to other

FDA-approved drugs, exhibiting a favorable toxicity profile and maintaining efficacy [116].

Rapamycin and derivatives (CCI-779 and RAD001) inhibit both mTOR and the downstream kinase target such as p70S6 kinase (p70S6K) and 4E-binding protein-1 (4E-BP1). The derivatives under clinical study have been shown to suppress the proliferation and growth of various tumor cell lines by blocking the G1-S transition in the cell cycle [117]. Furthermore, the immunosuppressant effect of rapamycin has been observed in several case studies, with transplanted patients reducing the incidence of cancer [118]. In ongoing clinical studies in prostate cancer in which the PI3K/Akt/mTOR pathway is highly expressed, it was observed that rapamycin and its derivatives were well tolerated in prostate cancer patients and decreased mTOR level [119]. In addition to the antiproliferative effect, RAD001 is also used as an immunosuppressant for the treatment of several malignancies in phase I study [120]. CCI779 that is the soluble ester of rapamycin [121] has been used for the treatment of several cancers in phase II study. This drug candidate has been used for T-cell leukemia, prostate, breast, and SCLC, as well as glioma and melanoma cell lines. CCI779 showed apoptosis induction, delaying the growth of the tumor, encouraging survival [105]. In combined treatment with apatinib, the treatment inhibits the proliferation and migration of small cell lung cancer cell lines [122].

Recently synthesized CYH33 is a novel PI3Kα inhibitor in phase 1b clinical trial for esophageal squamous cell carcinoma (ESCC) and breast cancer therapy. In vitro and in vivo studies show the anti-proliferative activity of this drug candidate to cell lines, induction of G1 phase arrest, and down-regulation of phosphorylated ERK in solid tumors [123]. The structure of all PI3K pathway inhibitors is shown in **Table 3**.

Target	Inhibitors		
PI3K	Idelalisib 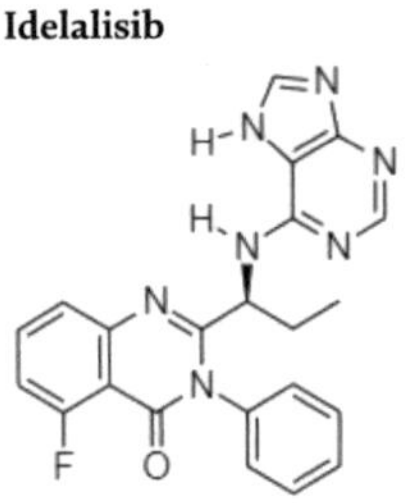	Copanlisib 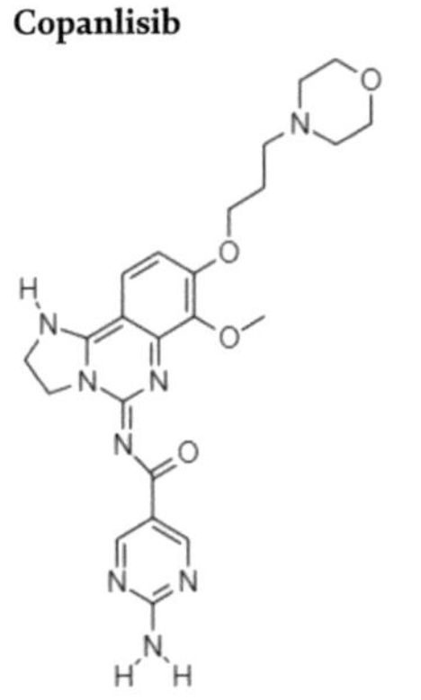	Rapamycin 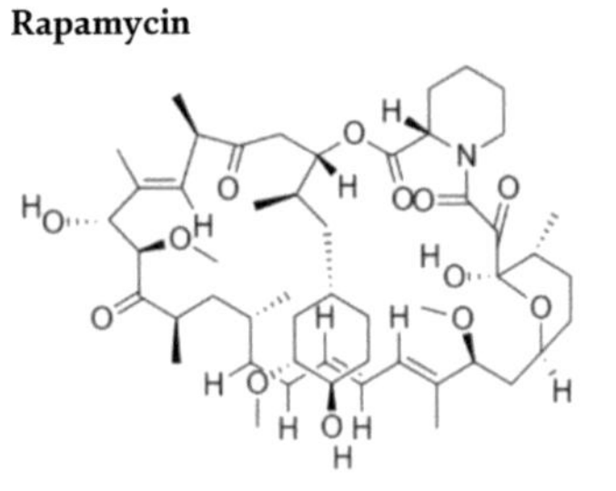
	CCI-779z 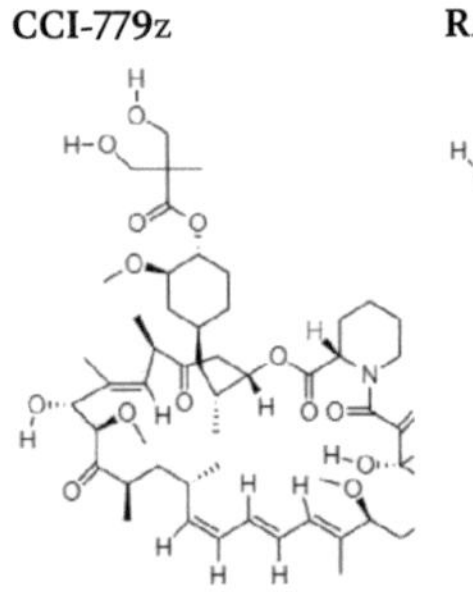	RAD001 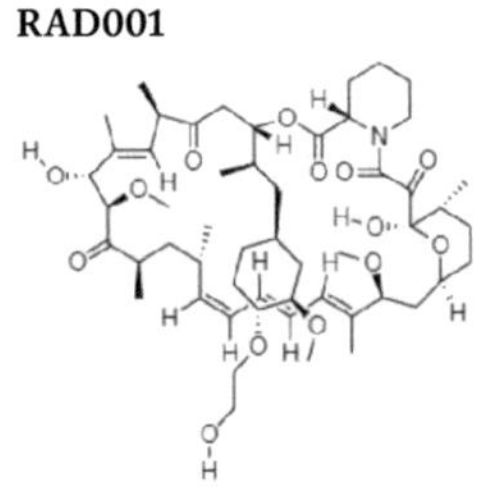	CYH33 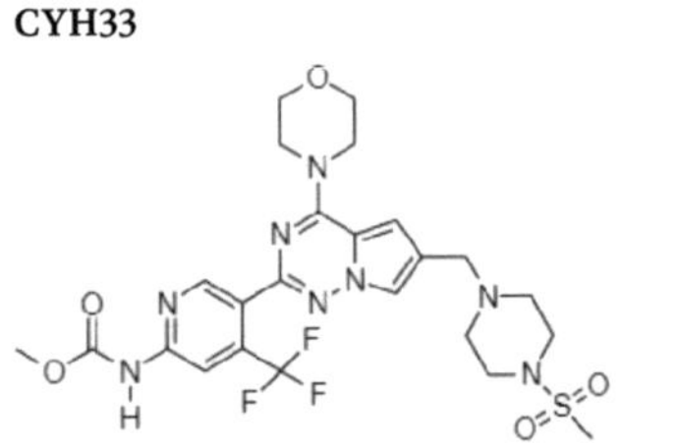

Table 3.
Structures of PI3K pathway inhibitors both in clinical development and FDA approved.

5. Cyclin-dependent kinase (CDK) inhibitors

CDKs found in a family of serine/threonine kinases are key regulators in the various phases of the cell cycle (**Figure 3**). CDKs ensure the continuation of the cell cycle by phosphorylating critical target proteins that are necessary to proceed to the next stage. Especially cells need to regulate the phosphorylation of kinases to sustain constant division in the presence of abnormal ploidy. Cyclin proteins, differently from CDKs, are synthesized at certain stages of the cell cycle. When the various cyclin form complexes with their target CDKs, it regulates the cell cycle transitions by enabling them to be phosphorylated and activated. For example, both cyclin D/CDK4 and cyclin D/CDK6 complexes direct phosphorylation of the Retinoblastoma gene (RB), which induces the separation of E2F to allow the transcription of the genes necessary for the proceed G1 to S phase transition. CDK inhibitors have been used in cancer therapy to interfere with the limitless replicative potential which is one of the hallmarks of cancer cells [124].

Palbociclib (PD 0332991) [128], Ribociclib (LEE011) [125], and Abemaciclib (LY2835219) [126] are novel dual inhibitors of both CDK4 and CKD6, that were approved by the FDA. Abemaciclib, more potent against CDK4 (IC50s of 2 nM for CDK4 and 10 nM for CDK6) [126]. These drugs have using for the treatment of postmenopausal women with HR-positive, HER2-negative advanced, or metastatic breast cancer. The action mechanism is that inhibiting the phosphorylation of Rb protein in the G1 phase results in cell cycle arrest [127]. Palbociclib has a synergistic effect in combination therapy with either letrozole or fulvestrant [128]. Abemaciclib also has a synergistic effect with gemcitabine [126].

BMS-387032 (SNS-032) is an aminothiazole, selectively designed for CDKs 2, 7, and 9 (with IC50s of 38 nM, 62 nM, and 4 nM, respectively) inhibition. Its activity was shown to inhibit both the cell cycle and the expression of anti-apoptotic proteins in various carcinoma models [129]. A phase I dose-escalation clinical trial study carried out to evaluate the safety, and clinical efficacy demonstrates limited clinical activity in heavily pretreated CLL and MM patients [130].

CYC202 (Seliciclib) shows potent inhibitors for broad CDK such as Cdk2, Cdk1, Cdk7, and Cdk9 (with IC50s of 0.1, 2.7, 0.5, and 0.8 mM, respectively), competing at their ATP binding sites [131]. This small molecule showed antitumor activity

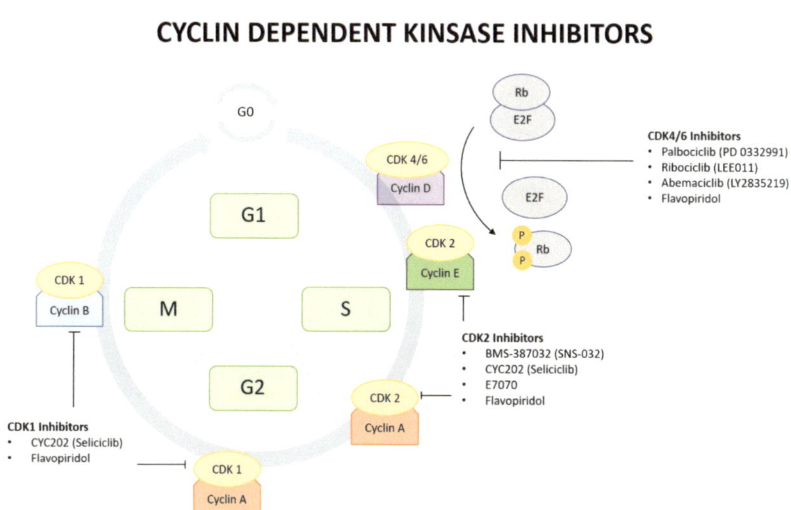

Figure 3.
Cyclin dependent kinases (CDKs) in the cell cycle and their inhibitors. CDKs are a family of serine/threonine kinases and key regulators in the cell cycle.

inducing apoptosis in multiple myeloma cell lines and has assayed in phase II study resulted in the dosing schedule being tolerable in nasopharyngeal carcinoma patients [132].

E7070 is a novel chloroindolyl-sulfonamide anticancer agent, which leads to induces arrest at the G1-S boundary and in company with mitigation in the expression of CDK2. E7070 has been assayed for melanoma cancer therapy in phase II and the results showed that CDK activity can be inhibited in tumor cells, but the dose and schedule applied are not suitable for single-agent chemotherapy for melanoma cancer treatment [133].

Flavopiridol has potent strong activity on several CDKs (CDK1, 2, 4, 6, and 7). In addition to controlling the cell cycle, it exhibits more than one action mechanism by showing an antiproliferative effect to leukemias and lymphoma cell lines

Target	Inhibitors		
CDK	**Palbociclib** 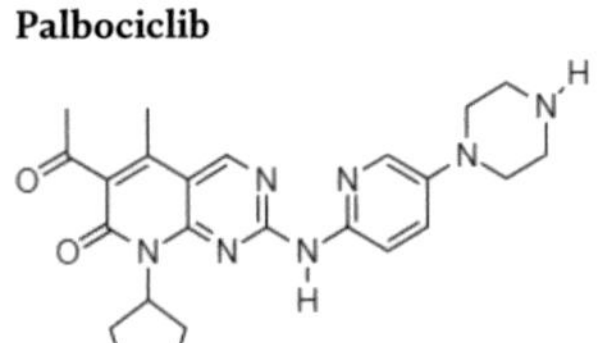	**BMS 387032** 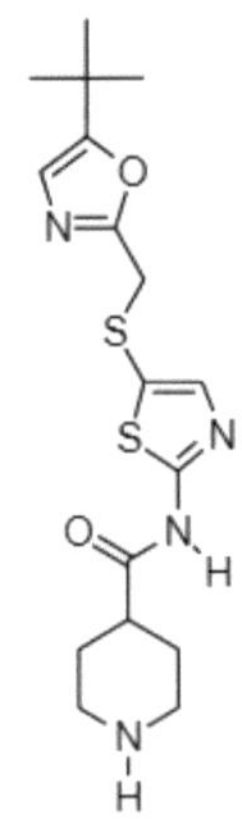	
	Ribociclib 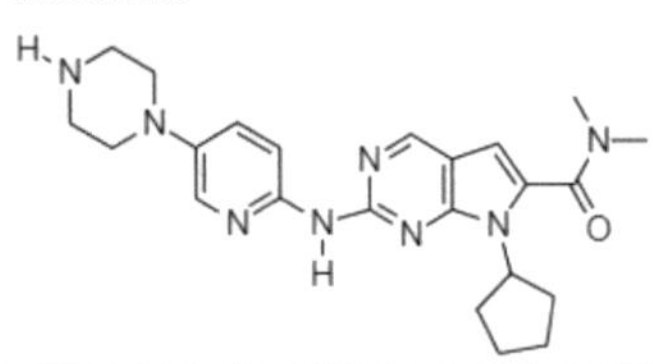		
	CYC202 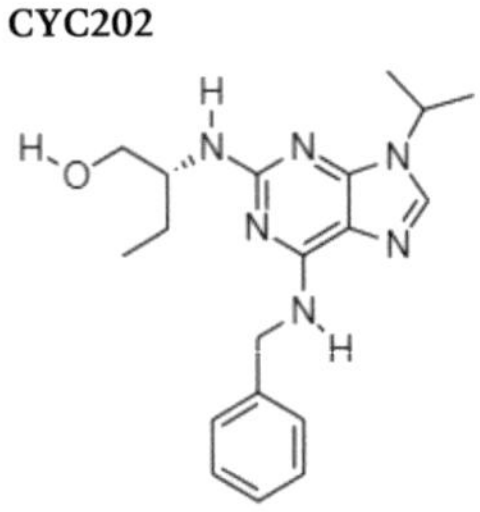	**E7070** 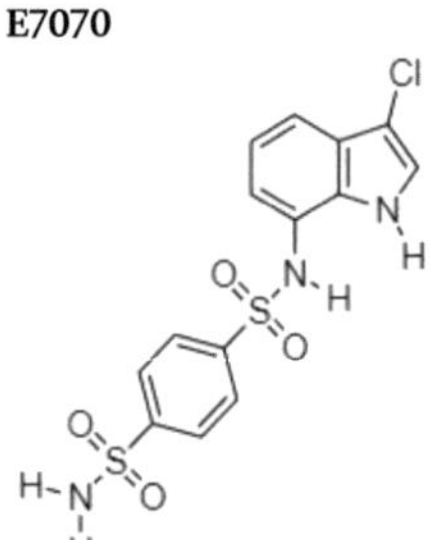	**Flavopiridol** 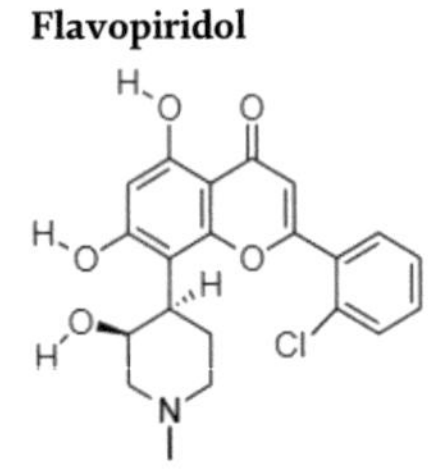
	Abemaciclib 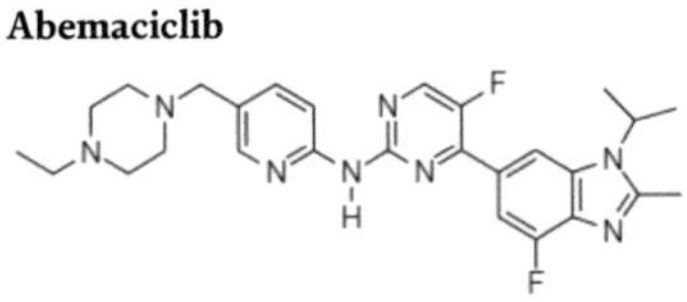		

Table 4.
Structures of CDK kinase inhibitors both in clinical development and FDA approved.

[134, 135]. Phase I and phase II studies have been tested on various progressive tumors and it has been observed that flavopiridol has no effect on metastatic renal carcinoma [135]. The structure of all CDK kinase inhibitors is shown in **Table 4**.

6. Other protein kinase inhibitors

Protein kinase C (PKC) is a family of serine/threonine kinases. They have important role in regulating a range of cellular functions including gene expression, differentiation, proliferation, cell cycle, apoptosis and cell migration. The PKC family includes 12 isoenzymes that can be divided into three groups depending on activation requirements. Conventional PKCs are calcium dependent and they require negatively charged phospholipid and diacylglycerol for activation. Novel PKCs are calcium independent, as conventional PKCs their activation requires phospholipid and diacylglycerol. Atypical PKCs are both calcium and diacylglycerol independent protein kinase group [136].

Regarding the PKC as a receptor for tumor-promoting phorbol esters, the researcher targets PKC for the potential treatment of cancer.

PKC is activated by phorbol esters and this event prevents cell death. Therefore, the inhibition of PKCα results in apoptosis. PKC activity has been reported to increase in many types of cancer, suggesting that PKC has important role in tumor formation. There are many PKC inhibitor candidates in clinical development for the treatment of cancer (**Figure 2**) [137].

First class of PKC inhibitors with anti-cancer activity are bryostatins. They are macrocyclic lactones extracted form marine bryozoan Bugula nerutina. Interaction of bryostatins with regulatory domain of PKC causes downregulation of the enzyme. Besides anti-proliferative, apoptotic and cytotoxic effects of Bryostatins on cancer cells, they also have immunomodulatory functions. Bryostatins provide the development of tumor-specific cytotoxic T-lymphocytes and stimulates the release of different cytokines such as TNF, IL-6. Both the immunomodulatory effect and downregulation of PKC has participated in antitumor effect of bryostatins [137, 138].

Second class of PKC inhibitors are staurosporines. Staurosporine is a microbial alkaloid derived from Streptomyces species organisms. In addition to PKC, staurosporine has shown the activity aganist different kinases including, pyruvate dehydrogenase kinase 1 (PDK1), PKA and PTK. Several staurosporines are under in clinical research such as UCN-01 (7-hydroxystaurosporine) or midostaurin (N-benzoyl staurosporine, PKC412) [138]. UCN-01 (7-hydroxy-staurosporine) has been reported to have more PKC inhibitory effects than staurosporine [105, 137]. UCN-01 causes cell cycle arrest in G1 step, thus leading the cell to death.

There is a growing interest in antisense therapy for PKC inhibitors. The structures of PKC inhibitors are shown in **Table 5**. ISIS 3521, an antisense therapy agent, is a phosphorothioate antisense oligodeoxynucleotide. ISIS 3521 binds to 3′ untranslated region (UTR) of human PKC-α messenger RNA (mRNA). This hybridization is then cleaved by RNase H and resulted in inhibition of PKC-α expression. Based on in vitro and in vivo studies results, ISIS 3521 may be a potential treatment agent for cancer patients [139].

Besides PKC inhibitor classes for cancer therapies described above, there are other agents including safingol, quercetin, antiestrogens, and miltefosine. Safingol is a synthetic sphingoid base analogue and safingol was the first to enter clinical trials. Quercetin belongs to flavonoids and widely distributed in nature. Quercetin inhibits different classes of protein kinases including PKC, phosphatidyl inositol-3 kinase. The PKC inhibitory effect of the classical antagonism of estradiol at the

Target	Inhibitors		
PKC	UCN-01 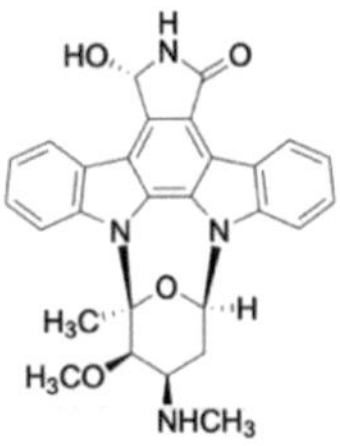	Bryostatin-1 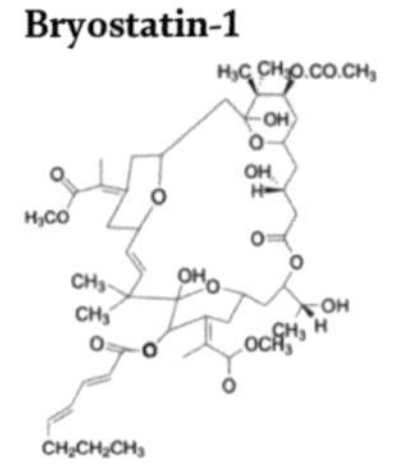	Staurosporine 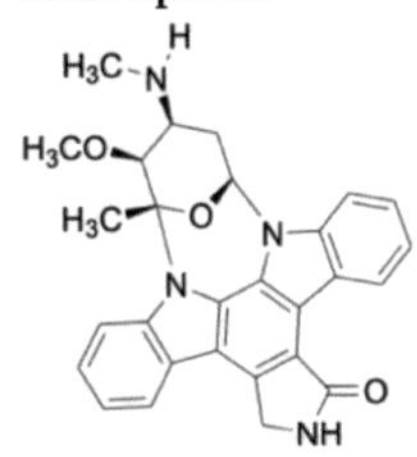
	Safingol 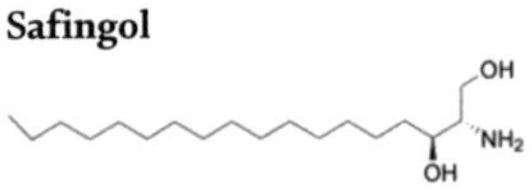	Miltefosine 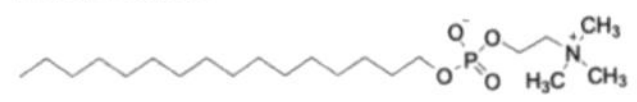	
	Ruboxistaurin 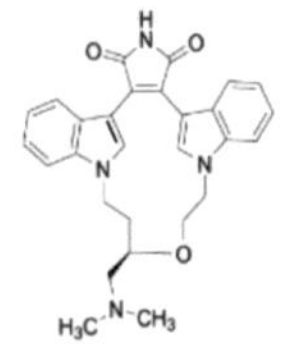	Tamoxifen 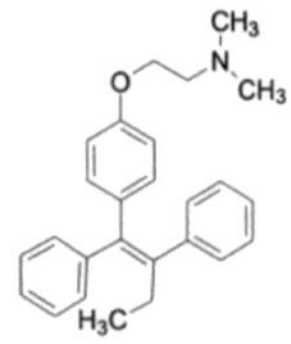	Quercetin 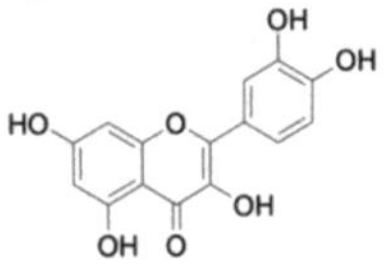

Table 5.
Structures of other kinases' inhibitors.

estrogen receptor level has been mentioned in many studies. However, the antiestrogen tamoxifen and its analogues have also been shown to inhibit PKC at very low concentrations. Miltefosine is an alkylphosphocholine and it shows its activation by preventing phospholipid metabolism. Miltefosine's antitumor activity is possibly associated with its abilitiy to inhibit PKC, but there has also been multiple alternative actions [137].

Although most protein kinase C inhibitors target the PKC-α, inhibitors targeting PKC-β have been investigated. PKC-β belongs to major PKC isoform classes. Hyperglycemia activated PKC-β leads to diabetic kidney diseases. LY333531 named as Ruboxistaurin selectively inhibits PKC-β. Recent studies showed that LY333531 significantly reduced PKC activity and PKC-β protein expression in the kidney [140, 141].

7. Conclusions

Protein kinases are potent oncogenes because of their ability to activate or inhibit other proteins. Furthermore, the ability to activate other protein kinases results in producing an exponential signal. In other words, a tiny signal can lead to a huge cellular response. This property of protein kinases makes their strict regulation crucial, and any dysregulation can lead to catastrophic outcomes. Many cancers are caused by the dysregulation of such oncogenic kinases, and inhibitors of those shown to increase overall survival in cancer patients. Although some tumors may gain resistance to some of those protein kinase inhibitors (PKIs), promising results of PKI administered cancer patients have led to developing new PKIs to treat PKI-related cancers [142].

Author details

Gizem Kursunluoglu[1,2], Duygu Erdogan[1,3], Elcin Cagatay[1,3], Esra Bulut Atalay[1,3], Seminay Guler[1,3], Yonca Gungor[1,3] and Hulya Ayar Kayali[1,3,4]*

1 İzmir Biomedicine and Genome (IBG) Center, İzmir, Turkey

2 Drug Application and Research Center, Erciyes University, Kayseri, Turkey

3 İzmir International Biomedicine and Genome Institute, Dokuz Eylul University, İzmir, Turkey

4 Faculty of Science, Department of Chemistry, Division of Biochemistry, Dokuz Eylul University, İzmir, Turkey

*Address all correspondence to: hulya.ayarkayali@gmail.com

References

[1] Johnson LN and Lewis RJ, Structural basis for control by phosphorylation. *Chemical Reviews*, 2001.101: p. 2209–42

[2] Manning G, Whyte DB, Martinez R, et al., The protein kinase complement of the human genome. *Science*, 2002. 298: p. 1912–34

[3] Wu, W., Cho, C., Lee, C., Fan, D., Wu, K., Yu, J., and Sung, J. (2010). Dysregulation of cellular signaling in gastric cancer. *Cancer Letters*, *295*(2), 144-153. DOI:10.1016/j.canlet.2010.04.025

[4] Ding, L., Wang, H., Lang, W., and Xiao, L. (2002). Protein Kinase C-ε Promotes Survival of Lung Cancer Cells by Suppressing Apoptosis through Dysregulation of the Mitochondrial Caspase Pathway. *Journal Of Biological Chemistry*, *277*(38), 35305-35313. DOI: 10.1074/jbc.m201460200

[5] Nadella, K., and Kirschner, L. (2005). Disruption of Protein Kinase A Regulation Causes Immortalization and Dysregulation of D-Type Cyclins. *Cancer Research*, *65*(22), 10307-10315. DOI:10.1158/0008-5472.can-05-3183

[6] Stehelin D, Varmus HE, Bishop JM, et al., DNA related to the transforming gene(s) of avian sarcoma viruses is present in normal avian DNA. *Nature*, 1976.260: p. 170–3

[7] Bitencourt, R., Zalcberg, I., and Louro, I. (2011). Imatinib resistance: a review of alternative inhibitors in chronic myeloid leukemia. Revista Brasileira De Hematologia E Hemoterapia, 33(6), 470-475. DOI: 10.5581/1516-8484.20110124

[8] Wieduwilt MJ, Moasser M. The epidermal growth factor receptor family: biology driving targeted therapeutics. Cellular and Molecular Life Sciences. 2008. 65(10): 1566-1584. DOI: 10.1007/s00018-008-7440-8.

[9] Hua H, Kong Q, Yin J, Zhang J, Jiang Y. Insulin-like growth factor receptor signaling in tumorigenesis and drug resistance: a challenge for cancer therapy. Journal of Hematology & Oncology. 2020. 13(1):64. DOI: 10.1186/s13045-020-00904-3.

[10] Tiash S, Chowdhury EH. Growth factor receptors: promising drug targets in cancer. Journal of Cancer Metastasis and Treatment. 2015. 1:190-200. DOI: 10.4103/2394-4722.163151.

[11] London M, Gallo E. Epidermal growth factor receptor (EGFR) involvement in epithelial-derived cancers and its current antibody-based immunotherapies. Cell biology international. 2020. 44(6): 1267-1282. DOI: 10.1002/cbin.11340.

[12] Lynch T J, Bell D W, Sordella R, Gurubhagavatula S, Okimoto R A, Brannigan BW, Harris PL, Haserlat SM, Supko JG, Haluska FG, Louis DN, Christiani DC, Settleman J, Haber DA. Activating mutations in the epidermal growth factor receptor underlying responsiveness of non–small-cell lung cancer to gefitinib. New England Journal of Medicine. 2004. 350(21): 2129-2139. DOI:10.1056/NEJMoa040938

[13] Pao W, Chmielecki J. Rational, biologically based treatment of EGFR-mutant non-small-cell lung cancer. Nature Reviews Cancer. 2010. 10(11): 760–74. DOI: 10.1038/nrc2947.

[14] Karachaliou N, Fernandez-Bruno M, Bracht JP, Rosell RJTCR. EGFR first- and second-generation TKIs—there is still place for them in EGFR-mutant NSCLC patients. Translational Cancer Research. 2018. 8:23-47. DOI: 10.21037/tcr.2018.10.06.

[15] Bartholomew C, Eastlake L, Dunn P, Yiannakis D. EGFR targeted therapy in lung cancer; an evolving story. Respiratory medicine case reports. 2017. 20: 137-40. DOI: 10.1016/j.rmcr.2017.01.016.

[16] Wu YL, Cheng Y, Zhou X, Lee KH, Nakagawa K, Niho S, Tsuji F, Linke R, Rosell R, Corral J, Migliorino MR, Pluzanski A, Sbar E, Wang T, White JL, Nadanaciva S, Sandin R, Mok TS. Dacomitinib versus geftinib as frst-line treatment for patients with EGFR-mutation-positive non-small-cell lung cancer (ARCHER 1050): a randomised, open-label, phase 3 trial. Lancet Oncology. 2017. 18(11):1454–66. DOI: 10.1016/S1470-2045(17)30608-3.

[17] Mok TS, Cheng Y, Zhou X, Lee KH, Nakagawa K, Niho S, Lee M, Linke R, Rosell R, Corral J, Migliorino MR, Pluzanski A, Sbar E, Wang T, White JL, Wu YL. Improvement in overall survival in a randomized study that compared dacomitinib with geftinib in patients with advanced non-small-cell lung cancer and EGFR-activating mutations. Journal of Clinical Oncology. 2018. 36(22):2244–50. DOI: 10.1200/JCO.2018.78.7994.

[18] Huang L, Jiang S, Shi Y. Tyrosine kinase inhibitors for solid tumors in the past 20 years (2001–2020). Journal of Hematology & Oncology. 2020. 13(1), 1-23. DOI: 10.1186/s13045-020-00977-0.

[19] Lim SM, Syn NL, Cho BC, Ross AS. Acquired resistance to EGFR targeted therapy in non-small cell lung cancer: Mechanisms and therapeutic strategies. Cancer Treatment Reviews. 2018. 65:1–10. DOI: 10.1016/j.ctrv.2018.02.006.

[20] Mok TS, Wu Y-L, Ahn M-J, Garassino MC, Kim HR, Ramalingam SS, Shepherd FA, He Y, Akamatsu H, Theelen WSME, Lee CK, Sebastian M, Templeton A, Mann H, Marotti M, Ghiorghiu S, Papadimitrakopoulou VA. Osimertinib or platinum-pemetrexed in EGFR T790M—positive lung cancer. New England Journal of Medicine. 2016. 376 (7):629–40. DOI: 10.1056/NEJMoa1612674.

[21] Reungwetwattana T, Nakagawa K, Cho BC, Cobo M, Cho EK, Bertolini A, Bohnet S, Zhou C, Lee KH, Nogami N, Okamoto I, Leighl N, Hodge R, McKeown A, Brown AP, Rukazenkov Y, Ramalingam SS, Vansteenkiste J. CNS response to osimertinib versus standard epidermal growth factor receptor tyrosine kinase inhibitors in patients with untreated EGFR-mutated advanced non-small-cell lung cancer. Journal of Clinical Oncology. 2018. 36 (33):3290–7. DOI: 10.1200/JCO.2018.78.3118.

[22] Lu S, Wang Q, Zhang G, Dong X, Yang C, Song Y, Chang G, Lu Y, Pan H, Chiu CH, Wang Z, Feng J, Zhou J, Xu X, Guo R, Chen J, Yang H, Chen Y, Yu Z, Shiah HS, Wang CC, Yang N, Fang J, Wang P, Wang K, Hu Y, He J, Wang Z, Shi J, Chen S, Wu Q, Sun C, Li C, Wei H, Cheng Y, Su WC, Hsia TC, Cui J, Sun Y, Yang JCH. A multicenter, open-label, single-arm, phase II study: the third generation EGFR tyrosine kinase inhibitor almonertinib for pretreated EGFR T790M-positive locally advanced or metastatic non-small cell lung cancer (APOLLO). Cancer Research. 2020 (80) (16 Supplement) CT190; DOI:10.1158/1538-7445.AM2020-CT190.

[23] Shi Y, Zhang S, Hu X, Feng J, Ma Z, Zhou J, Yang N, Wu L, Liao W, Zhong D, Han X, Wang Z, Zhang X, Qin S, Ying K, Feng J, Fang J, Liu L, Jiang Y. Safety, clinical activity, and pharmacokinetics of alfutinib (AST2818) in patients with advanced NSCLC with EGFR T790M mutation. Journal of Thoracic Oncology. 2020. 15(6):1015–26. DOI: 10.1016/j.jtho.2020.01.010.

[24] Shi Y, Fang J, Shu Y, Wang D, Yu H, Zhao Y, Zhang L, Zhu B, Li X, Chen G,

Shi J, Zheng R, Huang J, Yang S, Long J, Gao W, Greco M, Hu G, Li X. OA01.08 a phase I study to evaluate safety and antitumor activity of BPI-7711 in EGFRM+/T790M+ advanced or recurrent NSCLC patients. Journal of Thoracic Oncology. 2019. 14(11):1126–7. DOI: 10.1016/j.jtho.2019.09.022.

[25] Ahn M, Han J, Lee KH, Kim SW, Kim DW, Lee YG, Cho EK, Kim JH, Lee GW, Lee JS, Min YJ, Kim JS, Lee SS, Kim HR, Hong MH, Ahn JS, Sun JM, Kim HT, Lee DH, Kim S, Cho BC. Lazertinib in patients with EGFR mutationpositive advanced non-small-cell lung cancer: results from the dose escalation and dose expansion parts of a frst-in-human, open-label, multicentre, phase 1–2 study. The Lancet Oncology. 2019. 20(12):1681–90. DOI: 10.1016/S1470-2045(19)30504-2.

[26] Tan DSW, Leighl NB, Riely GJ, Yang JCH, Sequist LV, Wolf J, Seto T, Felip E, Aix SP, Jonnaert M, Pan C, Tan EY, Ko J, Moody SE, Kim DW. Safety and efcacy of nazartinib (EGF816) in adults with EGFR-mutant non-small-cell lung carcinoma: a multicentre, open-label, phase 1 study. The Lancet Respiratory Medicine. 2020. 8(6):561–72. DOI: 10.1016/S2213-2600(19)30267-X.

[27] Merla A, Goel S. Novel drugs targeting the epidermal growth factor receptor and its downstream pathways in the treatment of colorectal cancer: a systematic review. Chemotherapy research and practice, 2012.2012:387172. DOI: 10.1155/2012/387172.

[28] Cardoso F, Senkus E, Costa A, Papadopoulos E, Aapro M, Andre F, Harbeck N, Lopez BA, Barrios CH, Bergh J, Biganzoli L, Boers-Doets CB, Cardoso MJ, Carey LA, Cortés J, Curigliano G, Diéras V, El Saghir NS, Eniu A, Fallowfield L, Francis PA, Gelmon K, Johnston SRD, Kaufman B, Koppikar S, Krop IE, Mayer M, Nakigudde G, Offersen BV, Ohno S, Pagani O, Paluch-Shimon S, Penault-Llorca F, Prat A, Rugo HS, Sledge GW, Spence D, Thomssen C, Vorobiof DA, Xu B, Norton L, Winer EP. 4th ESOESMO International Consensus Guidelines for Advanced Breast Cancer (ABC 4). Annals of Oncology. 2018. 29 (8):1634–57. DOI: 10.1093/annonc/mdy192.

[29] Kannaiyan R, Mahadevan D. A comprehensive review of protein kinase inhibitors for cancer therapy. Expert review of anticancer therapy. 2018. 18 (12), 1249-1270. DOI: 10.1080/14737140.2018.1527688.

[30] Guo S, Colbert LS, Fuller M, Zhang Y, Gonzalez-Perez RR. Vascular endothelial growth factor receptor-2 in breast cancer. Biochimica et Biophysica Acta (BBA)-Reviews on Cancer. 2010; 1806: 108-121. DOI: https://doi.org/10.1016/j.bbcan.2010.04.004

[31] Li W, Feng C, Di W, Hong S, Chen H, Ejaz M, Yang Y, Xu TR. Clinical use of vascular endothelial growth factor receptor inhibitors for the treatment of renal cell carcinoma. European Journal of Medicinal Chemistry. 2020; 200:112482. DOI: https://doi.org/10.1016/j.ejmech.2020.112482

[32] Escudier B, Porta C, Schmidinger M, Rioux-Leclercq N, Bex A, Khoo V, Gruenvald V, Horwich A, ESMO Guidelines Committee. Renal cell carcinoma: ESMO clinical practice guidelines for diagnosis, treatment and follow-up. Annals of Oncology. 2016; 27: v58-v68. DOI: https://doi.org/10.1093/annonc/mdw328

[33] Llovet JM, Ricci S, Mazzaferro V, Hilgard P, Gane E, Blanc JF, Cosmo de Olivera A, Santoro A, Raoul JL, Forner A, Schwartz M, Porta C, Zeuzem S, Bolondi L, Greten TF, Galle PR, Seitz JF, Borbath I, Haussinger D, Giannaris T, Shan M, Moscovici M, Voliotis D, Bruix J. Sorafenib in advanced hepatocellular

carcinoma. The New England Journal of Medicine. 2008;359:378–90. DOI: https://doi.org/10.1056/nejmoa0708857

[34] Cheng A, Kang Y, Chen Z, Tsao CJ, Qin S, Kim JS, Luo R, Feng J, Ye S, Yang TS, Xu J, Sun Y, Liang H, Liu J, Wang J, Tak WY, Pan H, Burock K, Zou J, Voliotis D, Guan Z. Eficacy and safety of sorafenib in patients in the Asia-Pacifc region with advanced hepatocellular carcinoma: a phase III randomised, double-blind, placebo-controlled trial. Lancet Oncology. 2009; 10:25–34. DOI:https://doi.org/10.1016/s1470-2045(08)70285-7

[35] Bi F, Qin S, Gu S, Bai Y, Chen Z, Wang Z, Ying J, Lu Y, Meng Z, Pan H, Yang P, Zhang H, Chen X, Xu A, Liu X, Meng Q, Wu L, Chen F. Donafenib versus sorafenib as fIrst-line therapy in advanced hepatocellular carcinoma: An open-label, randomized, multicenter phase II/III trial. Journal of Clinical Oncology. 2020;38:4506-4506. DOI: 10.1200/JCO.2020.38.15_suppl.4506

[36] Bruix J, Qin S, Merle P, Granito A, Huang YH, Bodoky G, Pracht M, Yokosuka O, Rosmorduc O, Breder V, Gerolami R, Masi G, Ross PJ, Song T, Bronowicki JP, Hourmand IO, Kudo M, Cheng AL, Llovet JM, Finn RS, LeBerre MA, Baumhauer A, Meinhardt G, Han G. Regorafenib for patients with hepatocellular carcinoma who progressed on sorafenib treatment (RESORCE): a randomised, double-blind, placebo-controlled, phase 3 trial. Lancet. 2017;389:56–66. DOI: https://doi.org/10.1016/s0140-6736(16)32453-9

[37] Li Q, Qin S, Gu S, Chen X, Lin L, Wang Z, Xu A, Chen X, Zhou C, Ren Z, Yang L, Xu L, Bai Y, Chen L, Li J, Pan H, Cao B, FanG W, Yan P, Jin C. Apatinib as second-line therapy in Chinese patients with advanced hepatocellular carcinoma: a randomized, placebo-controlled, double-blind, phase III study. J Clin Oncol. 2020;38:4507-4507. DOI: 10.1200/JCO.2020.38.15_suppl.4507

[38] Abou-Alfa G,K Meyer T, Cheng AL, El-Khoueiry AB, Rimassa L, Ryoo BY, Cicin I, Merle P, Chen Y, Park JW, Blanc JF, Bolondi L, Klümpen HJ, Chan SL, Zagonel V, Pressiani T, Ryu MH, Venook AP, Hessel C, Borgman-Hagey AE, Schwab G, Kelley RK. Cabozantinib in patients with advanced and progressing hepatocellular carcinoma. The New England Journal of Medicine. 2018;379:54–63. DOI: https://doi.org/10.1056/nejmoa1717002

[39] Zhu AX, Finn RS, Ikeda M, Sung MW, Baron AD, Kudo M, Okusaka T, Kobayashi M, Kumada H, Kaneko S, Pracht M, Mamontov K, Meyer T, Mody K, Kubota T, Dutcus CE, Saito K, Siegel AB, Dubrovsky L, Llovet JM. A phase Ib study of lenvatinib (LEN) plus pembrolizumab (PEMBRO) in unresectable hepatocellular carcinoma (uHCC). Journal of Clinical Oncology. 2020;38: 4519-4519. DOI: 10.1200/JCO.2020.38.15_suppl.4519

[40] Han B, Li K, Wang Q, Zhang L, Shi J, Wang Z, Cheng Y, He J, Shi Y, Zhao Y, Yu H, Zhao Y, Chen W, Luo Y, Wu L, Wang X, Pirker R, Nan K, Jin F, Dong J, Li B, Sun Y. Efect of anlotinib as a third-line or further treatment on overall survival of patients with advanced non-small cell lung cancer: the ALTER 0303 phase 3 randomized clinical trial. JAMA OncolOGY. 2018;4:1569–75. DOI:https://doi.org/10.1001/jamaoncol.2018.3039

[41] Cheng Y, Wang Q, Li K, Shi J, Wu L, Han B, Chen G, He J, Wang J, Qin H, Li X. OA13.03 anlotinib as third-line or furtherline treatment in relapsed SCLC: a Multicentre, Randomized, Double-Blind Phase 2 Trial. Journal of Thoracic Oncology. 2018. 13(10): 351-352. DOI: 10.1016/j.jtho.2018.08.308

[42] Poddubskaya E, Baranova M, Allina D, Smirnov PY, Albert EA, Kirilchev AP, Aleshin AA, Sekacheva MI. Suntsova MV. Personalized prescription of tyrosine kinase inhibitors in unresectable metastatic cholangiocarcinoma. Experimental Hematology & Oncology. 2018. 7:21. DOI: 10.1186/s40164-018-0113-x.

[43] Sobhani N, Chumei F, Flores-Villanueva OP, Generali D, Li, Y. The fibroblast growth factor receptors in breast cancer: from oncogenesis to better treatments. International journal of molecular sciences. 2020. 21(6): 2011. DOI: 10.3390/ijms21062011.

[44] Vogel A, Sahai V, Hollebecque A, Vaccaro G, Melisi D, Al-Rajabi R, Paulson AS, Borad MJ, Gallinson D, Murphy AG, Oh D-Y, Dotan E, Catenacci DV, Van Cutsem E, Lihou CF, Zhen H, Féliz L, Abou-Alfa K. FIGHT-202: a phase II study of pemigatinib in patients (pts) with previously treated locally advanced or metastatic cholangiocarcinoma (CCA). Annals of Oncology. 2019. 30:v876. DOI: 10.1093/annonc/mdz394.031

[45] Javle M, Kelley RK, Roychowdhury S, Weiss KH, et al. AB051. P-19. A phase II study of infgratinib (BGJ398) in previously-treated advanced cholangiocarcinoma containing FGFR2 fusions. Hepatobiliary Surgery and Nutrition. 2019.8(Suppl 1): AB051. DOI: 10.21037/hbsn.2019.AB051

[46] Knowles MA, Hurst CD. Molecular biology of bladder cancer: new insights into pathogenesis and clinical diversity. Nature Reviews Cancer. 2015. 15(1):25–41. DOI: 10.1038/nrc3817

[47] Pal SK, Rosenberg JE, Hofman-Censits JH, Berger R, Quinn DI, et al. Efficacy of BGJ398, a Fibroblast Growth Factor Receptor 1-3 Inhibitor, in Patients with Previously Treated Advanced Urothelial Carcinoma with FGFR3 Alterations. Cancer Discovery. 2018. 8(7):812. DOI: 10.1158/2159-8290.CD-18-0229

[48] Bellmunt J, de Wit R, Vaughn DJ, Fradet Y, Lee J-L, Fong L, Vogelzang NJ, Climent MA, Petrylak DP, Choueiri TK, Necchi A, Gerritsen W, Gurney H, Quinn DI, Culine S, Sternberg CN, Mai Y, Poehlein CH, Perini RF, Bajorin DF. Pembrolizumab as secondline therapy for advanced urothelial carcinoma. The New England Journal of Medicine. 2017. 376(11):1015–26. DOI: 10.1056/NEJMoa1613683

[49] Haque S, Morris, JC. Transforming growth factor-β: A therapeutic target for cancer. Human vaccines & immunotherapeutics. 2017. 13(8): 1741-1750. DOI: 10.1080/21645515.2017.1327107

[50] Ma X, Cui Z, Du Z, Lin H. Transforming growth factor-β signaling, a potential mechanism associated with diabetes mellitus and pancreatic cancer?. Journal of cellular physiology. 2020. 235 (9):5882-5892. DOI: 10.1002/jcp.29605

[51] Hahn SA, Schutte M, Hoque AT, Moskaluk CA, da Costa LT, Rozenblum E, Weinstein CL, Fischer A, Yeo CJ, Hruban RH, Kern SE. DPC4, a candidate tumor suppressor gene at human chromosome 18q21.1. Science. 1996. 271(5247):350-3. DOI: 10.1126/science.271.5247.350

[52] Riggins GJ, Kinzler KW, Vogelstein B, Thiagalingam S. Frequency of Smad gene mutations in human cancers. Cancer Research. 1997. 57(13):2578-80.

[53] Halder SK, Beauchamp RD, Datta PK. Smad7 induces tumorigenicity by blocking TGF-beta-induced growth inhibition and apoptosis. Experimental Cell Research. 2005. 307(1):231-46. DOI: 10.1016/j.yexcr.2005.03.009

[54] Bruna A, Darken RS, Rojo F, Ocana A, Penuelas S, Arias A, Paris R,

Tortosa A, Mora J, Baselga J, Seoane J. High TGFbeta-Smad activity confers poor prognosis in glioma patients and promotes cell proliferation depending on the methylation of the PDGF-B gene. Cancer Cell. 2007. 11(2):147-60. DOI: 10.1016/j.ccr.2006.11.023

[55] Chod J, Zavadova E, Halaska MJ, Strnad P, Fucikova T, Rob L. Preoperative transforming growth factor-beta 1 (TGF-beta 1) plasma levels in operable breast cancer patients. European Journal of Gynaecological Oncology. 2008. 29(6):613-6. PMID: 19115689

[56] Fischer JR, Darjes H, Lahm H, Schindel M, Drings P, Krammer PH. Constitutive secretion of bioactive transforming growth factor beta 1 by small cell lung cancer cell lines. European Journal of Cancer. 1994. 30A (14):2125-9. DOI: 10.1016/0959-8049 (94)00364-B

[57] Labidi SI, Menetrier-Caux C, Chabaud S, Chassagne C, Sebban C, Gargi T, Biron P, Blay JY, Ghesquieres H. Serum cytokines in follicular lymphoma. Correlation of TGF-beta and VEGF with survival. Annals of hematology. 2010. 89(1):25-33. DOI: 10.1007/s00277-009-0777-8

[58] Langenskiold M, Holmdahl L, Falk P, Angenete E, Ivarsson ML. Increased TGF-beta 1 protein expression in patients with advanced colorectal cancer. Journal of Surgical Oncology. 2008. 97(5):409-15. DOI: 10.1002/jso.20961

[59] Shariat SF, Walz J, Roehrborn CG, Zlotta AR, Perrotte P, Suardi N, Saad F, Karakiewicz PI. External validation of a biomarker-based preoperative nomogram predicts biochemical recurrence after radical prostatectomy. Journal of Clınıcal Oncology. 2008. 26 (9):1526-31. DOI: 10.1200/JCO.2007.12.4669

[60] Shirai Y, Kawata S, Tamura S, Ito N, Tsushima H, Takaishi K, Kiso S, Matsuzawa Y. Plasma transforming growth factor-beta 1 in patients with hepatocellular carcinoma. Comparison with chronic liver diseases. Cancer. 1994. 73(9):2275-9. DOI: 10.1002/1097-0142(19940501)73:9<2275::AID-CNCR2820730907>3.0.CO;2-T

[61] von Rahden BH, Stein HJ, Feith M, Puhringer F, Theisen J, Siewert€ JR, Sarbia M. Overexpression of TGF-beta1 in esophageal (Barrett's) adenocarcinoma is associated with advanced stage of disease and poor prognosis. Molecular Carcinogenesis. 2006. 45(10):786-94. DOI: 10.1002/mc.20259

[62] Calon A, Lonardo E, Berenguer-Llergo A., Espinet E., Hernando-Momblona X., Iglesias M, Sevillano M, Palomo-Ponce S, Tauriello DVF, Byrom D, Cortina C, Morral C, Barceló C, Tosi S, Riera A, Attolini CSO, Rossell D, Sancho E, Batlle, E. Stromal gene expression defines poor-prognosis subtypes in colorectal cancer. Nature Genetics. 2015. 47(4): 320– U362. DOI: 10.1038/ng.3225

[63] Alsina-Sanchis E, Figueras A, Lahiguera A, Vidal A, Casanovas O, Graupera M, Villanueva A, Vinals, F. The TGF beta pathway stimulates ovarian cancer cell proliferation by increasing IGF1R levels. International Journal of Cancer. 2016. 139(8): 1894– 1903. DOI: 10.1002/ijc.30233

[64] Serova M, Tijeras-Raballand A, Dos Santos C, Muller N, Benhadji K, Paradis V, Faivre S, Raymond E, de Gramont A. Abstract 2094: Effects of TGF-beta signaling inhibition with LY2157299 in hepatocarcinoma models and in ex vivo whole tumor tissue samples from patient specimen. Cancer Research. 2013. 73(8 Suppl):nr 2094. DOI: 10.1158/1538-7445.AM2013-2094

[65] Ganapathy V, Ge R, Grazioli A, Xie W, Banach-Petrosky W, Kang Y,

Lonning S, McPherson J, Yingling JM, Biswas S, Mundy GR, Reiss M. Targeting the transforming growth factor-β pathway inhibits human basal-like breast cancer metastasis. Molecular cancer. 2010. 9(1): 1-16. DOI: 10.1186/1476-4598-9-122

[66] Zhang B., Halder SK, Kashikar ND, Cho Y-J., Datta A, Gorden, DL, Datta PK. Antimetastatic role of Smad4 signaling in colorectal cancer. Gastroenterology. 2010. 138(3): 969– U220. DOI: 10.1053/j.gastro.2009.11.004

[67] Ehata S, Hanyu A, Fujime M, Katsuno Y, et al. Ki26894, a novel transforming growth factor-beta type I receptor kinase inhibitor, inhibits in vitro invasion and in vivo bone metastasis of a human breast cancer cell line. Cancer Science. 2007. 98(1): 127– 133. 10.1111/j.1349-7006.2006.00357.x

[68] Shinto O, Yashiro M, Kawajiri H, Shimizu K, Shimizu T, Miwa A, Hirakawa, K. Inhibitory effect of a TGF beta receptor type-I inhibitor, Ki26894, on invasiveness of scirrhous gastric cancer cells. British Journal of Cancer. 2010. 102(5): 844– 851. DOI: 10.1038/sj.bjc.6605561

[69] Roddam AW, Allen NE, Appleby P, Key TJ, et al. Insulin like growth factors, their binding proteins, and prostate cancer risk: analysis of individual patient data from 12 prospective studies. Ann Intern Med. 2008. 149:461–71. DOI: 10.7326/0003-4819-149-7-200810070-00006

[70] Price AJ, Allen NE, Appleby PN, Crowe FL, et al. Insulin like growth factor-I concentration and risk of prostate cancer: results from the European Prospective Investigation into Cancer and Nutrition. Cancer Epidemiology, Biomarkers & Prevention. 2012. 21:1531–41. DOI: 10.1158/1055-9965.EPI-12-0481-T

[71] Ho GY, Zheng SL, Cushman M, Perez-Soler R, Kim M, Xue X, Wang T, Schlecht NF, Tinker L, Rohan TE, Wassertheil-Smoller S, Wallace R, Chen C, Xu J, Yu H. Associations of insulin and IGFBP-3 with lung cancer susceptibility in current smokers. Journal of the National Cancer Institute. 2016. 108(7). DOI: 10.1093/jnci/djw012

[72] Yoon YS, Keum N, Zhang X, Cho E, Giovannucci EL. Circulating levels of IGF-1, IGFBP-3, and IGF-1/IGFBP-3 molar ratio and colorectal adenomas: a meta-analysis. Cancer epidemiology. 2015. 39(6):1026-1035. DOI: 10.1016/j.canep.2015.09.004

[73] Chng WJ, Gualberto A, Fonseca R. IGF-1R is overexpressed in poor-prognostic subtypes of multiple myeloma. Leukemia. 2006. 20(1): 174-176. DOI: 10.1038/sj.leu.2403997

[74] Sprynski AC., Hose D, Kassambara A, Vincent L, Jourdan M, Rossi JF, Goldschmidt H., Klein B. Insulin is a potent myeloma cell growth factor through insulin/IGF-1 hybrid receptor activation. Leukemia. 2010. 24 (11): 1940-1950. DOI: 10.1038/leu.2010.192

[75] Vishwamitra D, George SK, Shi P, Kaseb AO, Amin HM. Type I insulin-like growth factor receptor signaling in hematological malignancies. Oncotarget. 2017. 8(1): 1814. DOI: 10.18632/oncotarget.12123

[76] Lin LH, Lin JS, Yang CC, Cheng HW, Chang KW, Liu CJ. Overexpression of platelet-derived growth factor and its receptor are correlated with oral tumorigenesis and poor prognosis in oral squamous cell carcinoma. International journal of molecular sciences. 2020. 21(7):2360. DOI: 10.3390/ijms21072360

[77] Kim S, You D, Jeong Y, Yoon SY, Kim SA, Lee J. E. Inhibition of platelet-derived growth factor receptor

synergistically increases the pharmacological effect of tamoxifen in estrogen receptor α positive breast cancer. Oncology Letters. 2006. 21(4): 1-8. DOI: 10.3892/ol.2021.12555

[78] Olson MF, Marais R. Ras protein signalling. Seminars in immunology. 2000;12:63-73. DOI: 10.1006/smim.2000.0208

[79] Boguski MS, McCormick F. Proteins regulating Ras and its relatives. Nature. 1993;366:643-654. DOI: 10.1038/366643a0

[80] Levitzki A. Protein kinase inhibitors as a therapeutic modality. Accounts of chemical research. 2003;36:462-469. DOI: 10.1021/ar0201207

[81] Davies H, Bignell GR, Cox C, Stephens P, Edkins S, Clegg S, et al. Mutations of the BRAF gene in human cancer. Nature. 2002;417:949-954. DOI: 10.1038/nature00766

[82] Pollock PM, Meltzer PS. Lucky draw in the gene raffle. Nature. 2002;417: 906-907. DOI: 10.1038/417906a

[83] Pruitt K, Der CJ. Ras and Rho regulation of the cell cycle and oncogenesis. Cancer letters. 2001;171: 1-10. DOI: 10.1016/s0304-3835(01)00528-6

[84] Bos JL. ras oncogenes in human cancer: a review. Cancer research. 1989; 49:4682-4689.

[85] Roskoski R, Jr. Properties of FDA-approved small molecule protein kinase inhibitors: A 2021 update. Pharmacological research. 2021;165: 105463. DOI: 10.1016/j.phrs.2021.105463

[86] Bagchi S, Rathee P, Jayaprakash V, Banerjee S. Farnesyl Transferase Inhibitors as Potential Anticancer Agents. Mini reviews in medicinal chemistry. 2018;18:1611-1623. DOI: 10.2174/1389557518666180801110342

[87] Wang Q, Chen F, Liu P, Mu Y, Sun S, Yuan X, et al. Scaffold-based analysis of nonpeptide oncogenic FTase inhibitors using multiple similarity matching, binding affinity scoring and enzyme inhibition assay. Journal of molecular graphics & modelling. 2021; 105:107898. DOI: 10.1016/j.jmgm.2021.107898

[88] Wang J, Yao X, Huang J. New tricks for human farnesyltransferase inhibitor: cancer and beyond. MedChemComm. 2017;8:841-854. DOI: 10.1039/c7md00030h

[89] Klochkov SG, Neganova ME, Yarla NS, Parvathaneni M, Sharma B, Tarasov VV, et al. Implications of farnesyltransferase and its inhibitors as a promising strategy for cancer therapy. Seminars in cancer biology. 2019;56: 128-134. DOI: 10.1016/j.semcancer.2017.10.010

[90] End DW, Smets G, Todd AV, Applegate TL, Fuery CJ, Angibaud P, et al. Characterization of the antitumor effects of the selective farnesyl protein transferase inhibitor R115777 in vivo and in vitro. Cancer research. 2001;61:131-137.

[91] Korzeniecki C, Priefer R. Targeting KRAS mutant cancers by preventing signaling transduction in the MAPK pathway. European journal of medicinal chemistry. 2021;211:113006. DOI: 10.1016/j.ejmech.2020.113006

[92] Lee HW, Sa JK, Gualberto A, Scholz C, Sung HH, Jeong BC, et al. A Phase II Trial of Tipifarnib for Patients with Previously Treated, Metastatic Urothelial Carcinoma Harboring HRAS Mutations. Clinical cancer research : an official journal of the American Association for Cancer Research. 2020; 26:5113-5119. DOI: 10.1158/1078-0432.CCR-20-1246

[93] Rao S, Cunningham D, de Gramont A, Scheithauer W, Smakal M, Humblet Y, et al. Phase III double-blind

placebo-controlled study of farnesyl transferase inhibitor R115777 in patients with refractory advanced colorectal cancer. Journal of clinical oncology : official journal of the American Society of Clinical Oncology. 2004;22:3950-3957. DOI: 10.1200/JCO.2004.10.037

[94] Whitehead RP, McCoy S, Macdonald JS, Rivkin SE, Neubauer MA, Dakhil SR, et al. Phase II trial of R115777 (NSC #70818) in patients with advanced colorectal cancer: a Southwest Oncology Group study. Investigational new drugs. 2006;24:335-341. DOI: 10.1007/s10637-005-4345-3

[95] Cohen SJ, Ho L, Ranganathan S, Abbruzzese JL, Alpaugh RK, Beard M, et al. Phase II and pharmacodynamic study of the farnesyltransferase inhibitor R115777 as initial therapy in patients with metastatic pancreatic adenocarcinoma. Journal of clinical oncology : official journal of the American Society of Clinical Oncology. 2003;21:1301-1306. DOI: 10.1200/JCO.2003.08.040

[96] Adjei AA, Mauer A, Bruzek L, Marks RS, Hillman S, Geyer S, et al. Phase II study of the farnesyl transferase inhibitor R115777 in patients with advanced non-small-cell lung cancer. Journal of clinical oncology : official journal of the American Society of Clinical Oncology. 2003;21:1760-1766. DOI: 10.1200/JCO.2003.09.075

[97] Baranyi M, Buday L, Hegedus B. K-Ras prenylation as a potential anticancer target. Cancer metastasis reviews. 2020; 39:1127-1141. DOI: 10.1007/s10555-020-09902-w

[98] Liu M, Bryant MS, Chen J, Lee S, Yaremko B, Lipari P, et al. Antitumor activity of SCH 66336, an orally bioavailable tricyclic inhibitor of farnesyl protein transferase, in human tumor xenograft models and wap-ras transgenic mice. Cancer research. 1998; 58:4947-4956.

[99] Feldkamp MM, Lau N, Roncari L, Guha A. Isotype-specific Ras·GTP-Levels Predict the Efficacy of Farnesyl Transferase Inhibitors against Human Astrocytomas Regardless of <em>Ras </em> Mutational Status. Cancer research. 2001;61:4425-4431.

[100] Morgillo F, Lee HY. Lonafarnib in cancer therapy. Expert opinion on investigational drugs. 2006;15:709-719. DOI: 10.1517/13543784.15.6.709

[101] Britten CD, Rowinsky EK, Soignet S, Patnaik A, Yao SL, Deutsch P, et al. A phase I and pharmacological study of the farnesyl protein transferase inhibitor L-778,123 in patients with solid malignancies. Clinical cancer research : an official journal of the American Association for Cancer Research. 2001;7: 3894-3903.

[102] Martin NE, Brunner TB, Kiel KD, DeLaney TF, Regine WF, Mohiuddin M, et al. A phase I trial of the dual farnesyltransferase and geranylgeranyltransferase inhibitor L-778,123 and radiotherapy for locally advanced pancreatic cancer. Clinical cancer research : an official journal of the American Association for Cancer Research. 2004;10: 5447-5454. DOI: 10.1158/1078-0432.CCR-04-0248

[103] Caponigro F, Casale M, Bryce J. Farnesyl transferase inhibitors in clinical development. Expert opinion on investigational drugs. 2003;12:943-954. DOI: 10.1517/13543784.12.6.943

[104] Leicht DT, Balan V, Kaplun A, Singh-Gupta V, Kaplun L, Dobson M, et al. Raf kinases: function, regulation and role in human cancer. Biochimica et biophysica acta. 2007;1773: 1196-1212. DOI: 10.1016/j.bbamcr.2007.05.001

[105] Dancey J, Sausville EA. Issues and progress with protein kinase inhibitors for cancer treatment. Nature reviews

Drug discovery. 2003;2:296-313. DOI: 10.1038/nrd1066

[106] Avruch J, Khokhlatchev A, Kyriakis JM, Luo Z, Tzivion G, Vavvas D, et al. Ras activation of the Raf kinase: tyrosine kinase recruitment of the MAP kinase cascade. Recent progress in hormone research. 2001;56: 127-155. DOI: 10.1210/rp.56.1.127

[107] Lyons JF, Wilhelm S, Hibner B, Bollag G. Discovery of a novel Raf kinase inhibitor. Endocrine-related cancer. 2001;8:219-225. DOI: 10.1677/erc.0.0080219

[108] Neuzillet C, Tijeras-Raballand A, de Mestier L, Cros J, Faivre S, Raymond E. MEK in cancer and cancer therapy. Pharmacology & therapeutics. 2014;141:160-171. DOI: 10.1016/j.pharmthera.2013.10.001

[109] Roberts PJ, Der CJ. Targeting the Raf-MEK-ERK mitogen-activated protein kinase cascade for the treatment of cancer. Oncogene. 2007;26: 3291-3310. DOI: 10.1038/sj.onc.1210422

[110] Lorusso PM, Adjei AA, Varterasian M, Gadgeel S, Reid J, Mitchell DY, et al. Phase I and pharmacodynamic study of the oral MEK inhibitor CI-1040 in patients with advanced malignancies. Journal of clinical oncology : official journal of the American Society of Clinical Oncology. 2005;23:5281-5293. DOI: 10.1200/JCO.2005.14.415

[111] Wang D, Boerner SA, Winkler JD, LoRusso PM. Clinical experience of MEK inhibitors in cancer therapy. Biochimica et biophysica acta. 2007; 1773:1248-1255. DOI: 10.1016/j.bbamcr.2006.11.009

[112] Fruman, D. A, Rommel C. PI3K and cancer: lessons, challenges and opportunities. Nature reviews Drug discovery. 2014; 13: 140-156. DOI: 10.1038/nrd4204

[113] Kannaiyan R, & Mahadevan, D. A comprehensive review of protein kinase inhibitors for cancer therapy. Expert review of anticancer therapy. 2018; 18: 1249-1270. DOI:10.1080/14737140.2018.1527688

[114] Markham, A. Idelalisib: first global approval. Drugs. 2014; 74: 1701-1707. DOI: 10.1007/s40265-014-0285-6

[115] O'Brien S M, Lamanna N, Kipps T J, Flinn I, Zelenetz A D, Burger J A, Coutre S E. A phase 2 study of idelalisib plus rituximab in treatment-naive older patients with chronic lymphocytic leukemia. Blood, The Journal of the American Society of Hematology. 2015; 126: 2686-2694. DOI: 10.1182/blood-2015-03-630947

[116] Dreyling M, Morschhauser F, Bouabdallah K, Bron D, Cunningham D, Assouline S E, Zinzani P L. Phase II study of copanlisib, a PI3K inhibitor, in relapsed or refractory, indolent or aggressive lymphoma. Annals of Oncology. 2017; 28: 2169-2178. DOI: 10.1093/annonc/mdx289

[117] Fasolo, A., Sessa, C. Current and future directions in mammalian target of rapamycin inhibitors development. Expert opinion on investigational drugs. 2011; 20: 381-394. DOI: 10.1517/13543784.2011.541154

[118] Lu, X., Paliogiannis, P., Calvisi, D. F., Chen, X. Role of the mammalian target of rapamycin pathway in liver cancer: from molecular genetics to targeted therapies. Hepatology, 2021; 73: 49-61. DOI: 10.1002/hep.31310

[119] Faes, S., Demartines, N., Dormond, O. Mechanistic Target of Rapamycin Inhibitors in Renal Cell Carcinoma: Potential, Limitations, and Perspectives. Frontiers in Cell and Developmental Biology. 2021; 9, 459. DOI: 10.3389/fcell.2021.636037

[120] Günther A, Baumann P, Burger R, Kellner C, Klapper W, Schmidmaier R,

Gramatzki, M. Activity of everolimus (RAD001) in relapsed and/or refractory multiple myeloma: a phase I study. Haematologica. 2015; 100(4), 541. DOI: 10.3324/haematol.2014.116269

[121] Dudkin L, Dilling M B, Cheshire P J, Harwood F C, Hollingshead M, Arbuck S G, Houghton, P J. Biochemical correlates of mTOR inhibition by the rapamycin ester CCI-779 and tumor growth inhibition. Clinical Cancer Research. 2001; 7: 1758-1764.

[122] Liu C, Zhang H, Li Y, Zhang Z, Shi R, Xu S, Chen J. Apatinib Combined with CCI-779 Inhibits the Proliferation and Migration of Small Cell Lung Cancer NCI-H446 Cells In Vitro. Zhongguo fei ai za zhi= Chinese Journal of Lung Cancer. 2020; 23: 216-222. DOI: 10.3779/j.issn.1009-3419.2020.104.08

[123] Xiang H Y, Wang X, Chen Y H, Zhang X, Tan C, Wang Y, Yang C H. Identification of methyl (5-(6-((4-(methylsulfonyl) piperazin-1-yl) methyl)-4-morpholinopyrrolo [2, 1-f] [1, 2, 4] triazin-2-yl)-4-(trifluoromethyl) pyridin-2-yl) carbamate (CYH33) as an orally bioavailable, highly potent, PI3K alpha inhibitor for the treatment of advanced solid tumors. European Journal of Medicinal Chemistry. 2018; 209: 112913. DOI: 10.1016/j.ejmech.2020.112913

[124] Asghar U, Witkiewicz A K, Turner N C, Knudsen E S. The history and future of targeting cyclin-dependent kinases in cancer therapy. Nature reviews Drug discovery. 2015; 14: 130-146. DOI: 10.1038/nrd4504

[125] Samson, K. LEE011 CDK Inhibitor Showing Early Promise in Drug-Resistant Cancers. Oncol. Times. 2014; 36, 39–40. DOI: 10.1097/01.COT.0000444043.33304.c1

[126] Gelbert L M, Cai S, Lin X, Sanchez-Martinez C, Del Prado M, Lallena M J, de Dios A. Preclinical characterization of the CDK4/6 inhibitor LY2835219: in-vivo cell cycle-dependent/independent anti-tumor activities alone/in combination with gemcitabine. Investigational new drugs. 2014; 32: 825-837. DOI: 10.1007/s10637-014-0120-7

[127] Łukasik P, Baranowska-Bosiacka I, Kulczycka K, Gutowska I. Inhibitors of Cyclin-Dependent Kinases: Types and Their Mechanism of Action. International Journal of Molecular Sciences. 2021; 22: 2806. DOI: 10.3390/ijms22062806

[128] Diéras V, Harbeck N, Joy A A, Gelmon K, Ettl J, Verma S, Finn R S. Palbociclib with letrozole in postmenopausal women with ER+/HER2− advanced breast cancer: hematologic safety analysis of the randomized PALOMA-2 trial. The oncologist. 2019; 24: 1514. DOI: 10.1634/theoncologist.2019-0019

[129] Nuwayhid S J, Hyde J, Aleshin A, Walker D H, Arkin M R. SNS-032 is a potent and selective inhibitor of CDK2, 7 and 9 and induces cell death by inhibiting cell cycle progression and the expression of antiapoptotic proteins. 2006

[130] Tong W G, Chen R, Plunkett W, Siegel D, Sinha R, Harvey R D, Wierda W G. Phase I and pharmacologic study of SNS-032, a potent and selective Cdk2, 7, and 9 inhibitor, in patients with advanced chronic lymphocytic leukemia and multiple myeloma. Journal of clinical oncology. 2010; 28: 3015. DOI: 10.1200/JCO.2009.26.1347

[131] McClue S J, Blake D, Clarke R, Cowan A, Cummings L, Fischer P M, Lane D P. In vitro and in vivo antitumor properties of the cyclin dependent kinase inhibitor CYC202 (R-roscovitine). International journal of cancer. 2002; 102: 463-468. DOI: 10.1002/ijc.10738

[132] Alsfouk A A, Alshibl H M, Altwaijry N A, Alsfouk B A, Al-Abdullah E S. Synthesis and biological evaluation of seliciclib derivatives as potent and selective CDK9 inhibitors for prostate cancer therapy. Monatshefte für Chemie-Chemical Monthly. 2021; 152:109-120. DOI: 10.1007/s00706-020-02727-x

[133] Smyth J F, Aamdal S, Awada A, Dittrich C, Caponigro F, Schöffski P, Punt C J A. Phase II study of E7070 in patients with metastatic melanoma. Annals of oncology. 2005; 16: 158-161. DOI: 10.1093/annonc/mdi016

[134] Sedlacek H, Czech J, Naik R, Kaur G, Worland P, Losiewicz M, Sausville E. Flavopiridol (L86 8275; NSC 649890), a new kinase inhibitor for tumor therapy. International journal of oncology. 1996; 9: 1143-1168. DOI: 10.3892/ijo.9.6.1143

[135] Sedlacek H H. Mechanisms of action of flavopiridol. Critical reviews in oncology/hematology. 2001; 38: 139-170. DOI: 10.1016/S1040-8428(00)00124-4

[136] Teicher BA. Protein Kinase C as a Therapeutic Target. Clinical cancer research. 2006;11:5336-45. DOI: 10.1158/1078-0432.ccr-06-0945

[137] Swannie HC, Kaye SB. Protein Kinase C Inhibitors. Current oncology reports. 2002;4:37-46. DOI: 10.1007/s11912-002-0046-7

[138] Cooke M, Magimaidas A, Casado-Medrano V, Kazanietz MG. Protein kinase C in cancer: The top Five Unanswered Questions. Molecular carcinogenesis. 2017;56:1531-1542. DOI: 10.1002/mc.22617

[139] Marshall JL, Eisenberg SG, Johnson MD, Hanfelt J, Dorr FA, El-Ashry D, Oberst M, Fuxman Y, Holmlund J, Malik S. A phase II trial of ISIS 3521 in patients with metastatic colorectal cancer. Clinical colorectal cancer. 2004;4: 268-274. DOI: 10.3816/ccc.2004.n.026

[140] Kunt T, Forst T, Kazda C, Harzer O, Engelbach M, Löbig M, Beyer J, Pfützner A. The beta-specific protein kinase C inhibitor ruboxistaurin (LY333531) suppresses glucose-induced adhesion of human monocytes to endothelial cells in vitro. Journal of diabetes science and technology. 2007;6: 929-935. DOI: 10.1177/193229680700100620

[141] Yonggui W, Guozhong W, Xiangming Q, Hui L, Hao Q, Jijia S, Shantan L. Protein Kinase C β Inhibitor LY333531 Attenuates Intercellular Adhesion Molecule-1 and Monocyte Chemotactic Protein-1 Expression in the Kidney in Diabetic Rats. Journal of Pharmacological Sciences. 2006;4: 335-343. DOI: 10.1254/jphs.FP0050896

[142] Kumari, A., Silakari, O., & Singh, R. (2018). Recent advances in colony stimulating factor-1 receptor/c-FMS as an emerging target for various therapeutic implications. Biomedicine & Pharmacotherapy, 103, 662-679. doi: 10.1016/j.biopha.2018.04.046